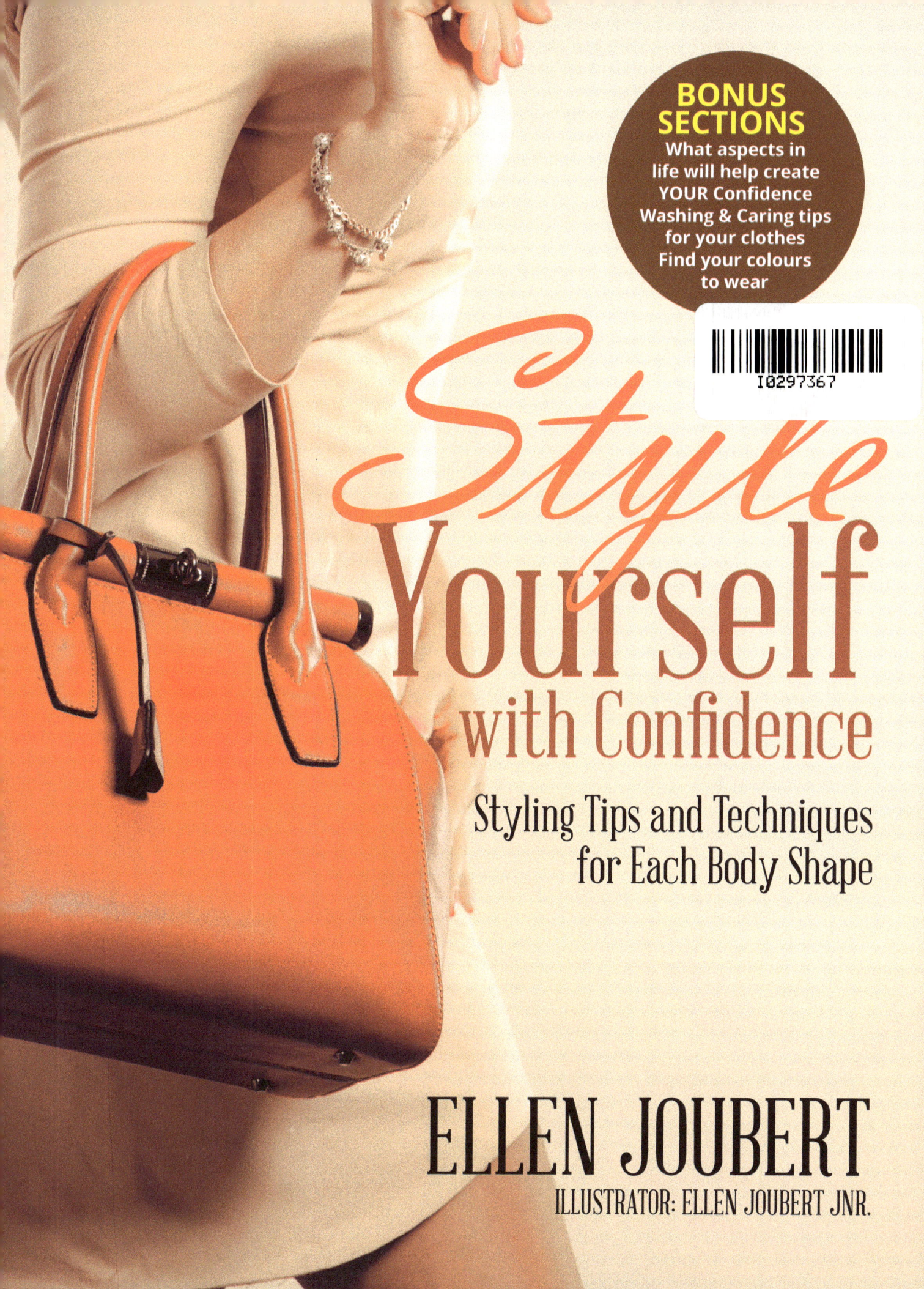

BONUS SECTIONS
What aspects in life will help create YOUR Confidence
Washing & Caring tips for your clothes
Find your colours to wear

Style Yourself with Confidence

Styling Tips and Techniques for Each Body Shape

ELLEN JOUBERT
ILLUSTRATOR: ELLEN JOUBERT JNR.

Copyright © 2019 by Ellen Joubert.

Published by Leading Voice International Pty Ltd

All rights reserved. No part of this book may be reproduced in any written, electronic, recording, or photocopying without written permission of the publisher or author. The exception would be in the case of brief quotations embodied in the critical articles or reviews and pages where permission is specifically granted by the publisher or author.

Although every precaution has been taken to verify the accuracy of the information contained herein, the author and publisher assume no responsibility for any errors or omissions. No liability is assumed for damages that may result from the use of information contained within.

Rev. date: 31/05/2019

ISBN:

Softcover 978-0-6485691-2-1
Hardcover 978-0-6485691-3-8
Ebook 978-0-6485691-4-5

I dedicate this book to all the women who are looking for a practical application to dress themselves with confidence. A woman, who has gained an overall professional and confident look, will experience the amazing doors that will open in her personal and professional life.

Women need to celebrate who they are and realize they have a very important role to play in the world. They have the power to change the direction of the world because they have an influence on their family, their friends, their work colleagues, and especially their children. A confident woman will help the people around her to be more confident in life. Confident individuals are usually happier and healthier, believe in themselves more, will not want to harm others, will stand up for themselves, will not allow any wrongdoing against others, and achieve greater success in life.

I salute all women! If you are a girl, or a young woman, or a mother, or a grandmother, you are special, and you have to realize it.

Foreword

I grew up in life without any shortage, but I really wished I could buy the clothes I wanted without having to look at the price tag. I've always admired women who can afford beautiful boutique and branded clothing; they just come across as so beautiful and professional.

In my late teens and early twenties, I completed a diploma in beauty technology in South Africa. My desire then was to know everything necessary on how to make myself beautiful. Another door opened for me to complete a modelling course at an international modelling academy. Together these two qualifications helped birth a modelling and deportment school. I trained children from three years to young adults in their late twenties on how to walk on the catwalk, on how to look their best, and on how to gain more confidence. The results were remarkable during the nineties where shy individuals turned into these beautiful and confident personalities. My desire (and it still is today) is to give the youth and all women the tools and knowledge on how to improve their appearance and to grow their self-confidence. To have self-confidence today is really necessary to achieve success in life. Self-confidence is the key for more opportunities to present themselves, and it also gives a sense of self-worth to the individual.

Through the years of studying, attending seminars, and personal experiences, I realized that there is no ugly person on this earth. The only problem is that some people never had the opportunity to learn the tricks on how to dress their best and grooming techniques. From my own experiences and what I have seen, the majority of married women and mums tend to put themselves last on the list and actually refrain from spoiling themselves. Alternatively, a person loses focus and puts someone else or others first. We put our husbands and children first in everything. It is sometimes as if some women think that they do not deserve something because they are the mother and needs to provide, which is the right thing to do, because if we brought children into this life, it is our responsibility to look after them as best we can, till they are confident and prepared to go out into the world and start their own life. There is also no problem in blessing our children and husbands. The saying 'Whatever you sow, you will reap' has proven to be true. In other words, if you sow potatoes, you cannot expect corn to grow; and if you sow hate, you cannot expect love to be the end result. What I want to bring across to each woman is that we must not look after everyone else around us and let ourselves be run to the ground. If you are already a mum or still a teenager on your way to being a mum one day, always remember to groom yourself in a way that will earn you respect, especially after you've had a child or children.

It is crucial that we women look after ourselves and keep ourselves beautiful and positive throughout our lifetime, not just for ourselves, but also for our family members. I have read a story once where a husband and wife signed a contract when they got married that they would keep themselves beautiful and have the same weight throughout their marriage, as the day they got married. At first I thought that it was unreasonable to sign a contract like that. Women have children, which changes their body shape forever, and of course, as we all get older, our bone structure, skin, and hair also change. After thinking and reviewing it in my mind over and over again, I realized that it was not such an unreasonable request at all. It is irrational to think that we have to look the same thirty years after our marriage. But what I think we can take away from this story is, we should take care of our body in such a way that we can be the best version of ourselves at any point and time during our lifetime.

How many young women spend a lot of time and money on themselves to look beautiful so that they can catch their dream husband, but after the marriage and having a couple of kids, are just not as focused on themselves anymore? Generally, this is when a woman's focus shifts to their children, forgetting about themselves. Of course after we are born, we grow into strong young adults (around twenty-one to twenty-five years), which then changes the clock against us, and we start to age quicker from thereon. So much more reason why we have to spend time to preserve ourselves for longer. It is so beautiful when a woman ages gracefully, don't you think?

There are so many ways to age gracefully when it comes to looking after your skin, getting dressed, applying make-up, and living healthy. The purpose of this book is to show women there are more in getting dressed every day than just jumping into a tracksuit to clothe oneself. My desire is that the explanations and examples in this book will help you to think for yourself. It is easy to follow instructions in a book on how to dress if you are a certain body shape, but what I want for you to understand is the reasoning behind the suggestions; not only for you to understand certain recommendations, but also to work it out for yourself from now on. And you will be the role model and style trainer for your daughters, and they in turn for their daughters.

As you read through this book, you will realize that it does not cost extravagantly to dress stylishly. It only takes some guidance and common sense after finishing this book. There are so many different styling techniques, which I am sure will change as life continues. Most of the examples in this book, I believe, are timeless and can be used for decades to come. There may be add-ons to the different styling tips, but most concepts in this book will always create the same effect no matter what. For example, I will describe turn-ups on trousers later in this book, it says that turn-ups will make legs look shorter because of the horizontal line created at the seam line; therefore, it is best for short women with shorter legs to avoid turn-ups on their trousers, which will make them appear shorter. It is okay, though, for tall women with long legs to wear turn-ups on their trousers, as it will break the length and their legs will appear shorter. This technique also falls in the optical illusion section, where we trick the eye with clever ways in appearing shorter or taller. Read more about optical illusion tricks in the 'How to Create Optical Illusion with Style' section.

My wish is that all women who read this book will become confident in themselves by knowing how to use style to look their best and subsequently love themselves. These two concepts will change your world into a more positive experience. When women become confident, they will be confident mothers, and ultimately their children will become confident. When the information learned in this book are passed on, future generations will have a beautiful appearance and be confident.

You are welcome to contact me and give your feedback on how you found the information in this book.

Ellen Joubert

Your partner in style and confidence

Acknowledgements

Firstly, I want to thank God, who has ordered my every step since I was born and enabled me to have the time to write this book. Secondly, I want to thank my family, who supported me all the way on the journey in writing this book—my husband, Marius; dad, Johan; daughters, Maria and Ellen (Junior). Thank you for your encouragement. I love you all!

Thanks to my daughter Ellen (Junior), who was alongside me every step of the way, assisting me with her creative skills as a graphic designer, drawing images, creating new images, and giving me professional advice. Without your help, Ellen, the task would have been enormous. So thank you for your support and love in bringing this book to life.

Thanks to my long-time friend in Australia, Adele, from *Adele Miles Photography*, who helped me take the photos in the mix-and-match ideas section and our profile photo.

Thanks to Kim Innes, owner of *Kimbo's Fashions* in Midland, Western Australia; for allowing us using clothes from her boutique, to show some mix-and-match ideas. Also thanks to Mekene Lomutopa for being our model in the mix-and-match ideas section.

God bless!

Ellen Joubert

Wife, daughter, mother, and friend

Contents

First Impressions and the Art of Being Well-Dressed 9
    First Impressions 10
    The Art of Being Well-Dressed 11
    The Meaning of Being Stylish, Fashionable, and Trendy 12

The 75-25 Per Cent Principle in Wardrobe Planning and Mix-and-Match Ideas 14
    The 75-25 Per Cent Principle in Wardrobe Planning 15
    Examples of Mix-and-Match Wardrobes 21

Fashion and Body Proportions 26
    Fashion and Body Proportions 27
    The Three Body Types 30
    The Scale of Body Shapes and Sizes 31
    The Eight Different Body Shapes 33
    Style Personalities 37

Line-, Symmetrical-, Asymmetrical Designs And Creating Optical Illusion with Line Design 39
    Line Design 40
    Symmetrical and Asymmetrical Designs 42
    Creating Optical Illusion with Line Design 45

The Best Necklines for Each Face Shape and Body Shape 48
    Necklines and Face Shapes 49
    The Different Garment Necklines 53

Shoulder Lines and Creating Optical Illusion with Style 70
    Creating Balance with Shoulder Lines 71
    How to Create Optical Illusion with Style 76

Styling Tips for the Different Body Shapes to Create Balance 85
    Rectangle Body Shape 86
    Inverted Triangle or Heart Body Shape 88

- Hourglass Body Shape 90
- Round/Apple Body Shape 92
- Triangle/Pear Body Shape 94
- Petite Body Shape 96
- Lean Body Shape 98
- Plus-Size Body Shape 100

Choosing the Right Shoes 103
- How to Choose Your Shoes 104
- How do you Clean Shoes 108
- Walking in High Heels 111

Find Your Colours 113
- Find Your Perfect Colours to Wear 114
- The Four Colour Seasons 119
- Flow Colour Analysis 126
- The Twelve Flow Seasons 129
- Get to Know the Colour Wheel 154

Prescription- and Sunglasses Frames for Each Face Shape 155
- Choose the Best Frame for Your Face Shape 156

Washing and Caring for Your Clothes...163
- The Best Washing and Caring Techniques for Your Clothes 164
- Ironing Your Clothes...171
- The Best Ironing Sequence 173

Building Your Self-Confidence 175
- What is Self-Confidence? 177
- Dealing with Bullying 179
- Healthy Relationships 181
- Easy Steps to Help You Gain Your Self-Confidence 182
- Characteristics of Love 183
- Final Note... 184
- My Quick Reference Guide 186
- Bibliography 190

First Impressions and the Art of Being Well-Dressed

First Impressions

When it comes to how we dress, the one important fact to know is that people have always and will continue to judge us on our appearance. We make decisions about people within the first three to seven seconds of meeting them. That is why it is fair to say, we only get one chance to make a good first impression. To be well-dressed, will earn you respect, and can actually make you more successful in life.

We live in a judgemental world, where people are quick to make assumptions and categorize individuals based on what they see.

The meaning of the term *well-dressed* is to be attired in clothing that is of good quality, is properly fitted, and is appropriate and becoming.

Does that mean we always have to look like we are stepping out of a fashion magazine? No, of course not!

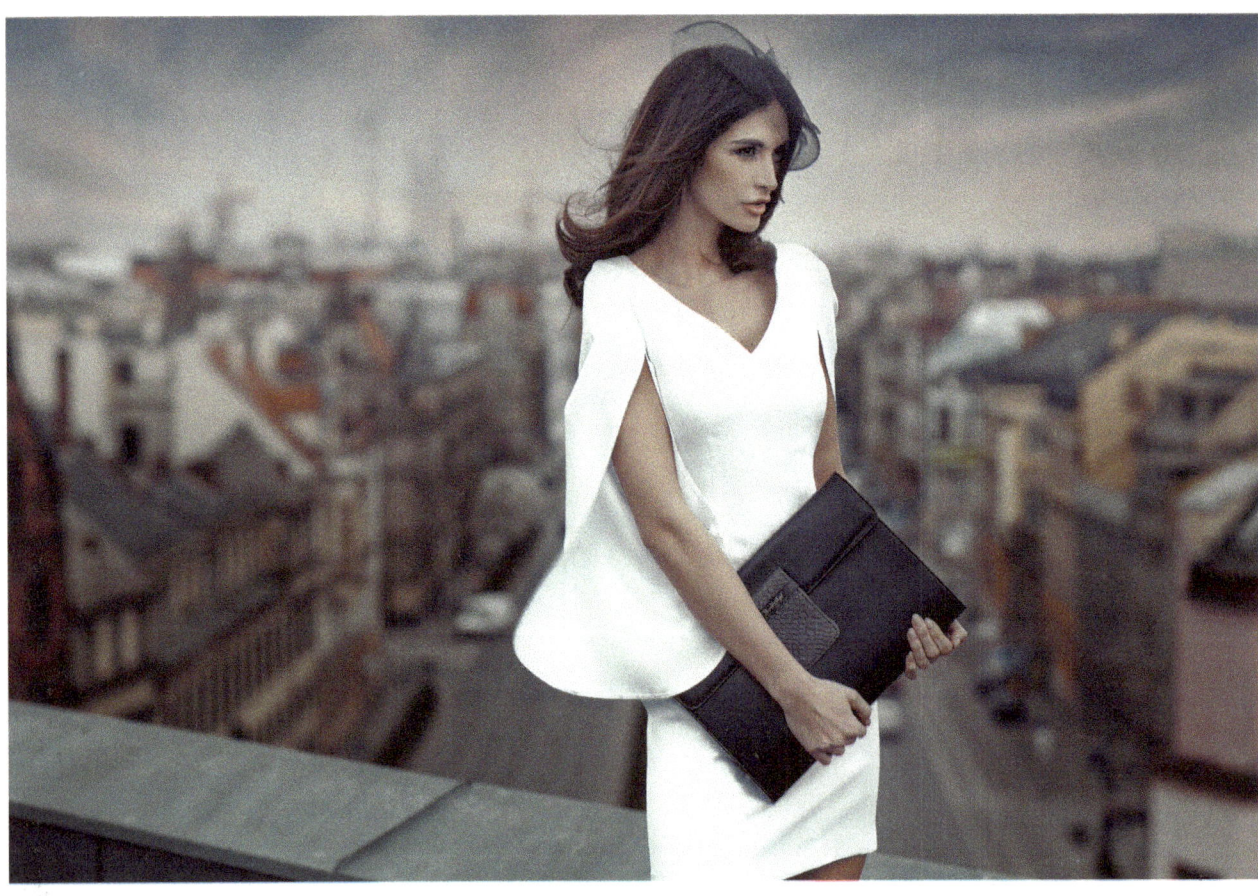

The Art of Being Well-Dressed

The benefits of being well-dressed:

- Well-dressed women stand out from a crowd and attract good attention.
- Dressing well gives a woman confidence. A young woman who has confidence and believes in herself, will rise to the challenge and achieve greater success in life.
- A well-dressed woman stands a better chance at getting a professional job than someone who does not care how they look.

To most, good styling does not come naturally. We are not born with good-style genes. Fashion stores and magazines are a great help to show us which garments and colours work well together. A lot of times, we wear what we see around us and what looks good on others. The reason why it works is not always apparent.

This book will help you gain the knowledge on how to dress your specific features the best, which will give you so much more confidence and makes it easier when buying clothes. Once you have the understanding on how clothing styles and colour work, you'll be enlightened for the rest of your life, and be able to help not only yourself but others too. You'll be a role model for your children and even your grandchildren.

The good news is that you do not have to buy your clothes only at high-end boutiques to make a good lasting impression. Even the most extravagant outfit can make you look tired and dull when the style and colours do not fit your features. Less-expensive brands can be worn stylishly when the suggestions in this book are followed. We are never too young or too old to learn about style and how to dress correctly according to our own body shape.

Our aim in life must be to be stylish. "Being stylish" is not the same as "being fashionable" or "being trendy". It can be a waste of money when we only buy trendy or fashionable clothes, because fashion comes and fashion goes. Being stylish will last a lifetime. Dressing well shows maturity and also radiates an image of self-respect and self-worth.

Being well-dressed is to pursue the following statements:

- Wear clothes that fit you well. Extra-large may feel comfortable, but wearing clothes a size or two too big, or vice versa, does not do justice. Tight fitted clothes, on the other hand, can reveal any unattractive contours a body might have, while oversized clothes can make you look bigger.
- Clothes must be clean and free from stains, tears, rips, and creases, unless the fabric creates creases and rips as a fashion statement.
- Colour combinations of clothing pieces must be colour-coordinated. For example, blue and brown do not work well together, pink and green do not work well together either, etc. I'll explain more on colour in the 'Find Your Colours' section of this book.

- Find your personal style. Perceive your body shape and skin tone to work out which styles and colours will suit you best. Your body type and shape should always take preference over fashion trends.
- Bra straps and underwear must not be exposed with any outfit.
- Dress for the occasion. Jeans and T-shirts are a common sight today and are accepted in many locations. The problem is, they do not rise above these social norms.
- Choose clothing styles that compliment your personality. Do you like sporty, classic, natural, creative, contemporary, or dramatic styles?
- Wear quality underwear that enhances your body shape. Replace with new underwear every couple of years or when necessary to keep having a beautiful shape.
- Shoes must fit the outfit and occasion. For example, do not wear high heels that are uncomfortable if you have to walk long distances.
- Never walk with high heels when the heels are worn out, the clicking sounds are awful, and it will have lost its style. Rather get the heels repaired if it's your favourite pair.
- Dressing your age is important, mothers must not try and dress like their teenage daughters.

The Meaning of Being Stylish, Fashionable, and Trendy

Being Stylish

Being stylish means that you show elegance, taste, and refinement. The outfit suits your body shape, personality, skin tone, and it is current. Therefore, a person looks attractive.

Being Fashionable or Trendy

Being fashionable or trendy simply means that you're following the latest trends in fashion.

The Risks of Following Fashion or Trends Slavishly

Not all fashion trends will fit with all the different body shapes perfectly. Therefore, a lot of women may not look attractive and fashionable at the same time. Some styles can make one woman look amazing, while the same style will make another look dull or unattractive. That is why we must not confuse stylish with fashionable or trendy.

Four Essentials of Looking Stylish

1. The style of your outfit must fit your body shape.
2. The style of your outfit must suit your personality.
3. The colour(s) of the outfit must fit your skin tone and features.
4. The outfit must be current and not dating back ten to twenty years, unless the specific fashion made a comeback.

The 75-25 Per Cent Principle in Wardrobe Planning and Mix-and-Match Ideas

The 75-25 Per Cent Principle in Wardrobe Planning

It is wise to create your wardrobe on the 75-25 per cent principle. Stock your wardrobe with 75 per cent stylish clothes that are mostly in plain colours and not too colourful; they should easily fit with colourful shirts, jackets, shawls, shoes, and handbags. Choose pieces in your personal colours that will fit well together. Stylish means something that has a plain design that will be in for many years. For example, corporate-style skirts, trousers, and jackets.

The other 25 per cent should be fashionable or trendy pieces that are current. Current means that your clothing style still fits in or are close to the fashion of the specific time you are wearing them, and does not date back a decade or two. The other recommendation is to create a mix-and-match wardrobe that will allow you to design more different looks than only having garment sets. Rather than buying ten dresses or having ten sets that cannot be mixed-and-matched, it is better to have the option of mixing-and-matching, which will maximize your wardrobe.

Mix-and-Match Ideas

How to style twelve clothing pieces into thirty different looks:

- two dresses
- one skirt
- one pair of trousers
- four colourful shirts
- one sleeveless vest, long or short
- three jackets (it can be long, short- or three-quarter-sleeved jackets that are corporate or leather and in colours that will fit with all the other garments' colours, for example, black, brown, navy blue, or deep beige).

1. One pair of trousers with four different shirts = four looks.
2. One pair of trousers with four different shirts and sleeveless vest = four looks.
3. One pair of trousers with four different shirts and long sleeve jacket = four looks.
4. One skirt with four different shirts = four looks.
5. One skirt with four different shirts and sleeveless vest = four looks.
6. One skirt with four different shirts and long sleeve jacket = four looks.
7. Dress number 1 by itself = one look.
8. Dress number 1 with two different jackets = two looks.

9. Dress number 2 by itself = one look.
10. Dress number 2 with a long sleeve jacket and vest = two looks.

With accessories like scarfs, handbags, and shoes, you can add more looks.

The following twelve clothing pieces are used to explain how to mix-and-match.

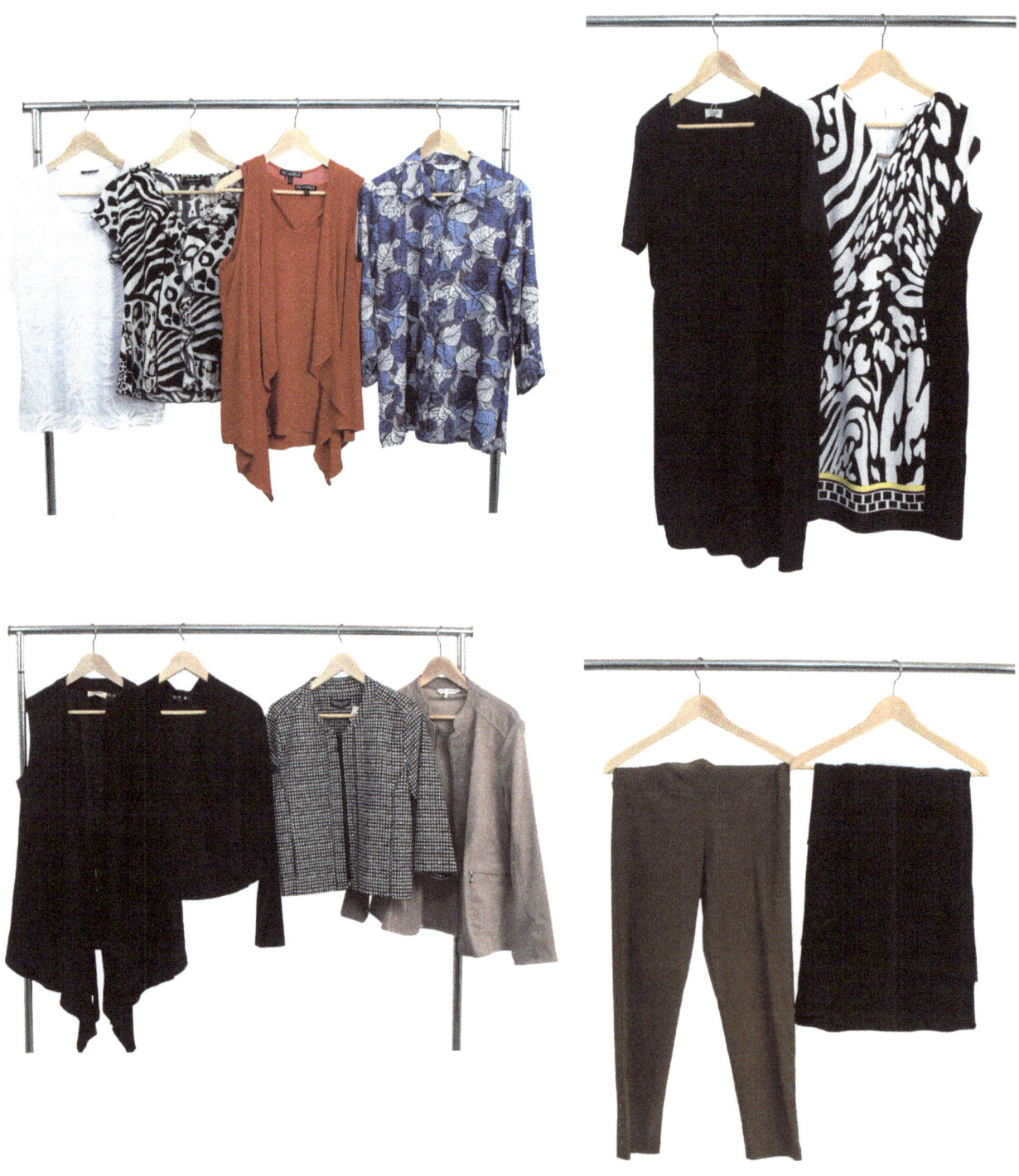

Four Different Styling Looks: Trousers with Four Different Shirts

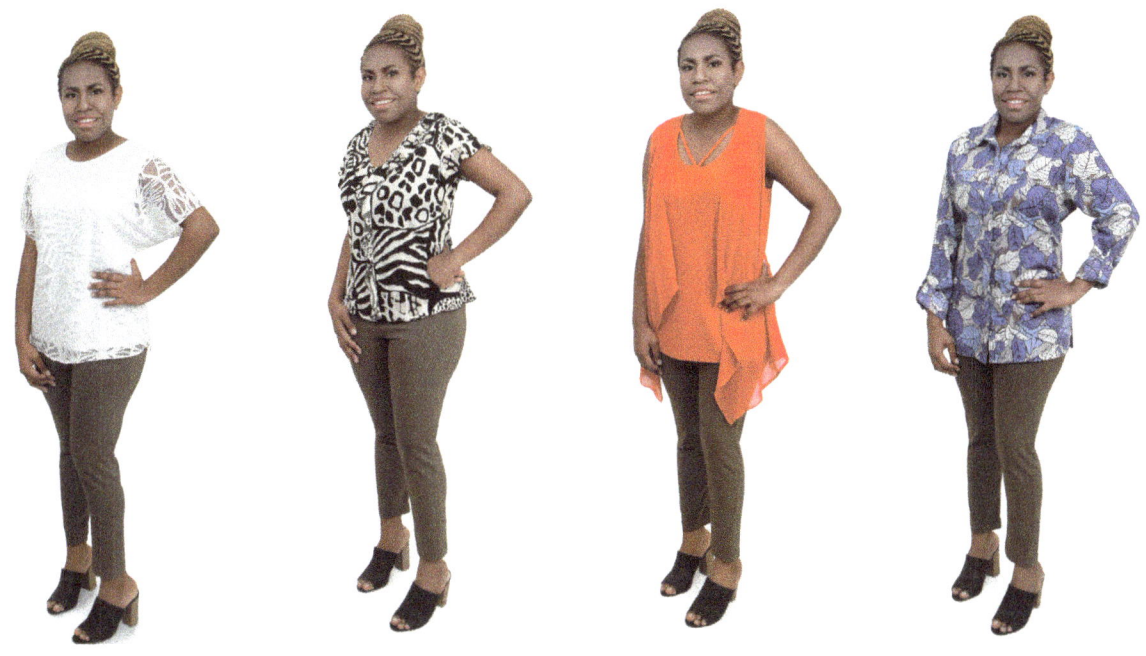

Four Different Styling Looks: Skirt with Four Different Shirts

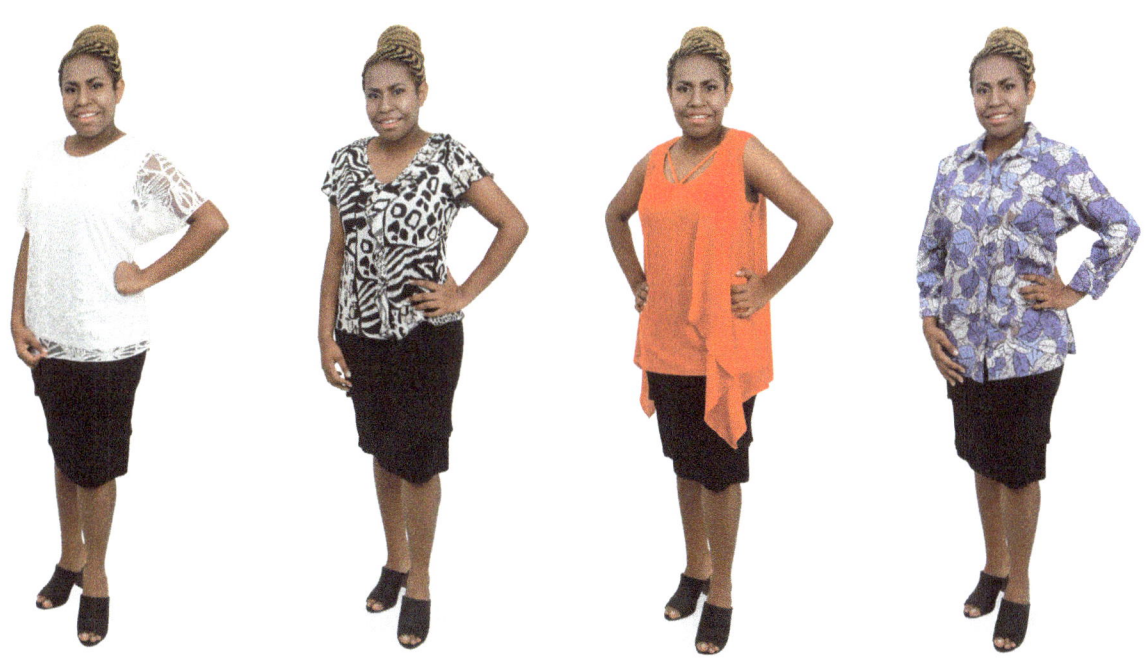

Four Different Styling Looks: Trousers with Four Different Shirts and Vest

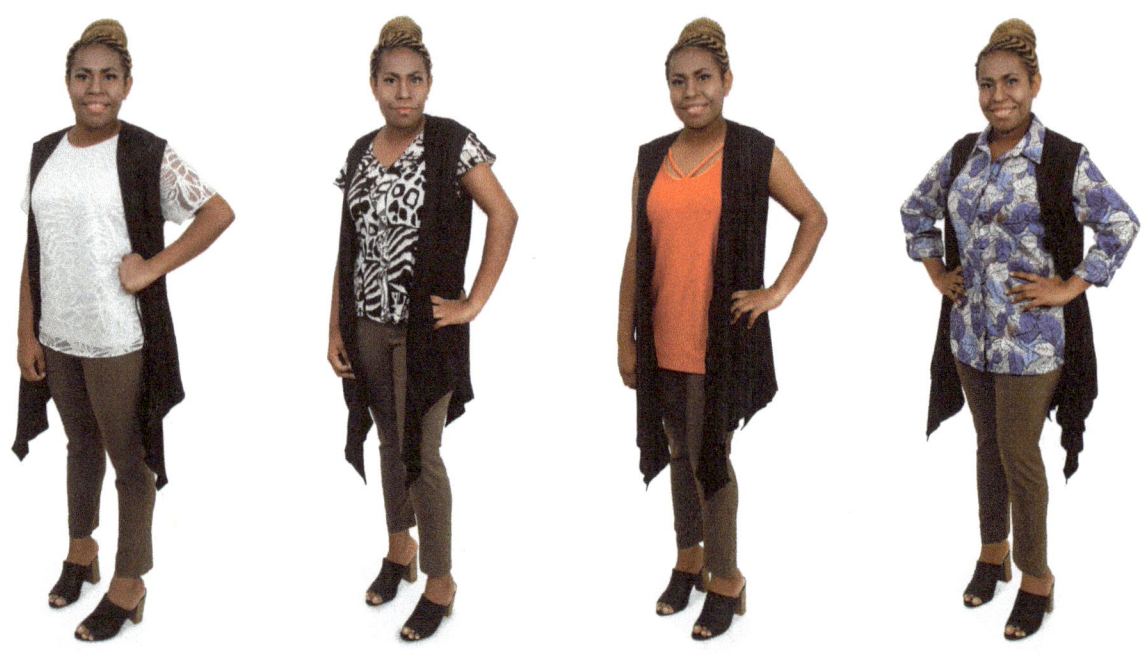

Four Different Styling Looks: Trousers with Four Different Shirts and Long Sleeve Jacket

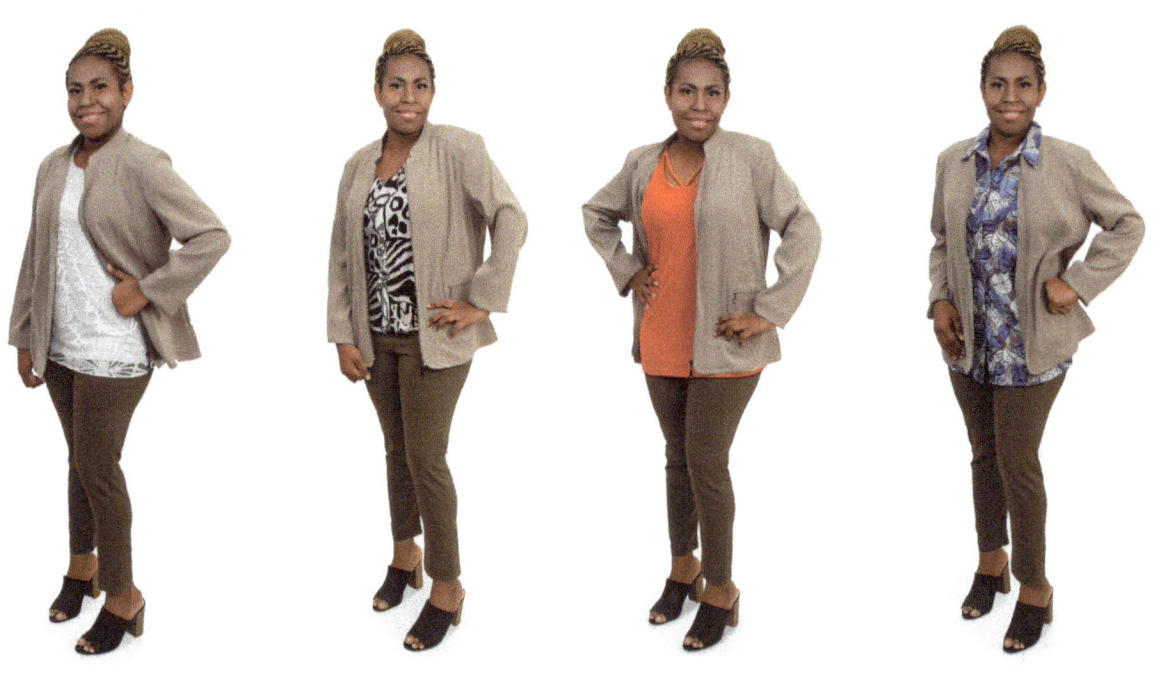

Four Different Styling Looks: Skirt with Four Different Shirts and Vest

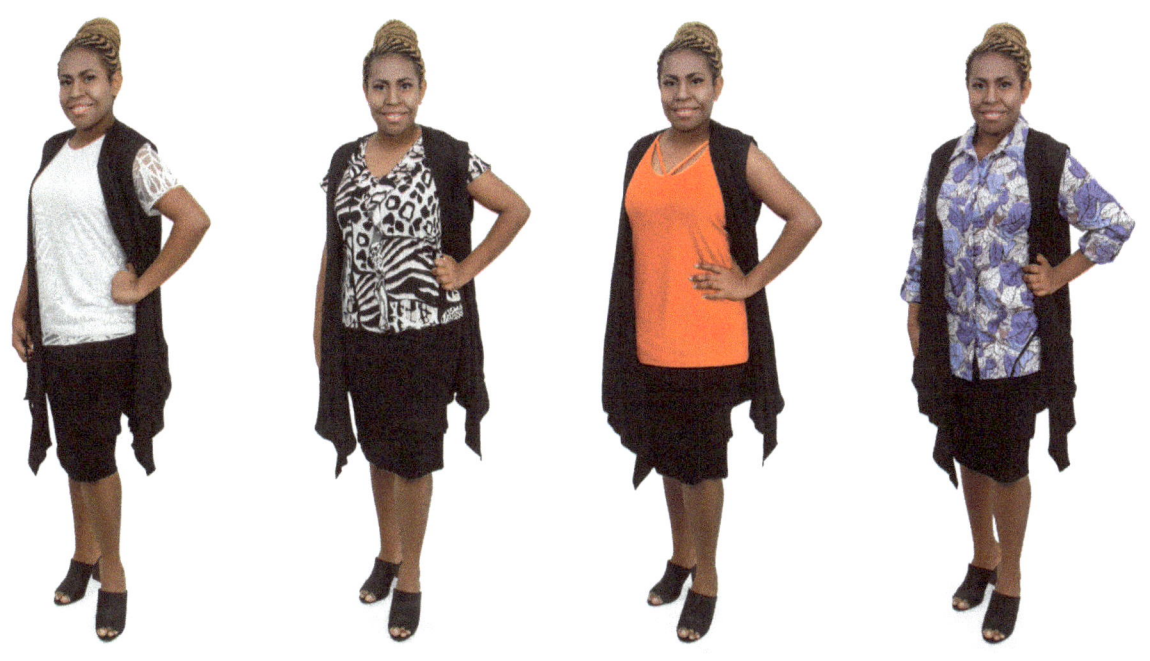

Four Different Styling Looks: Skirt with Four Different Shirts and Long Sleeve Jacket

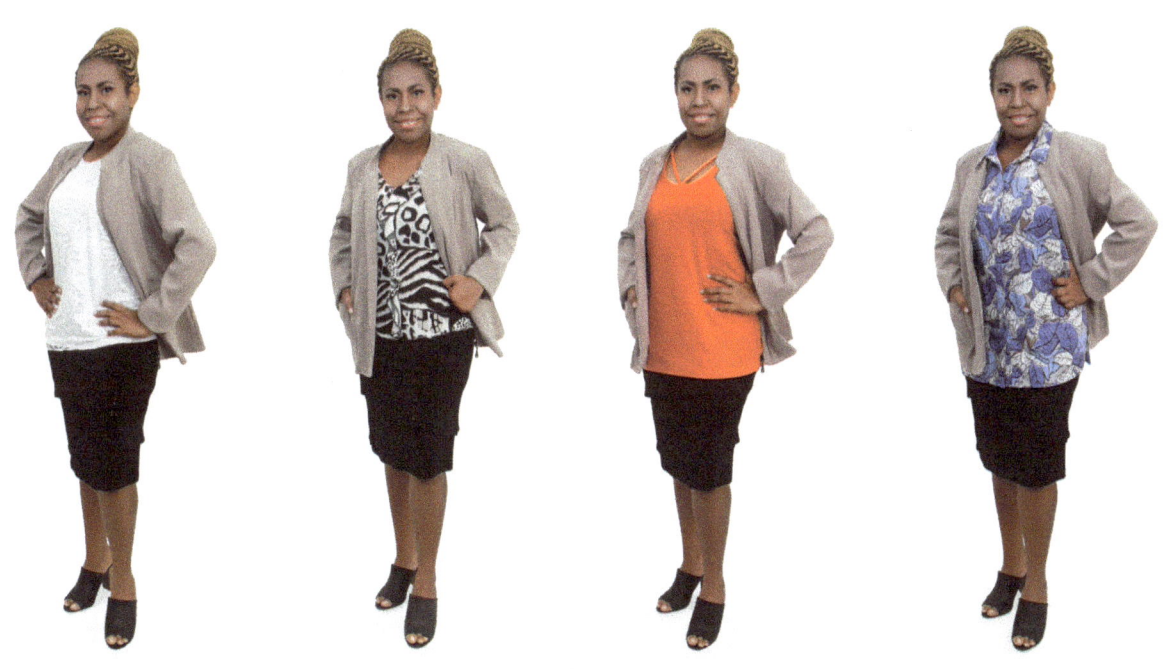

Three Different Styling Looks: Dress Number 1 by itself and Two Jackets

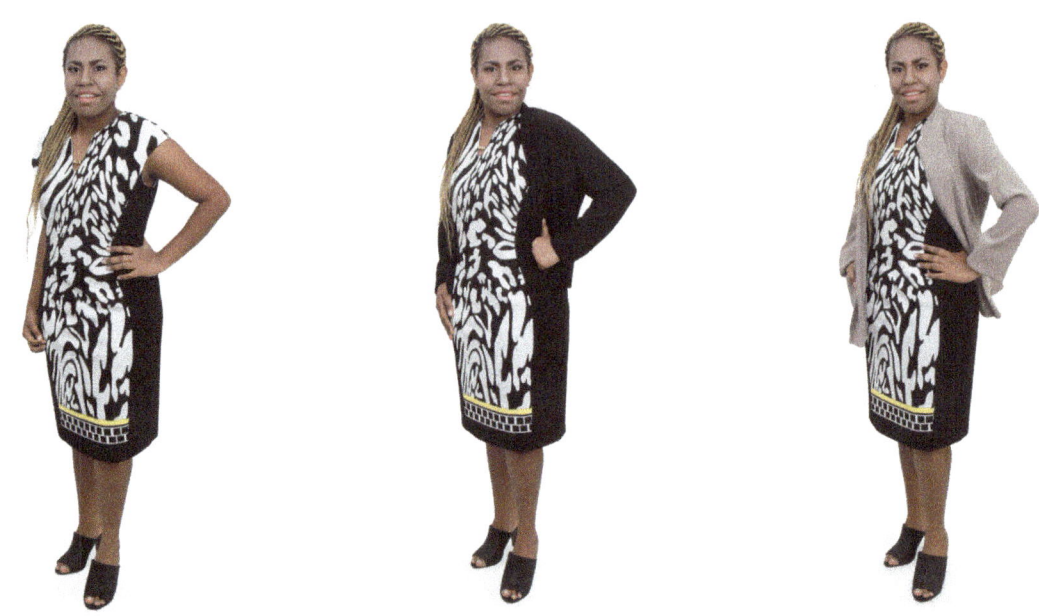

Three Different Styling Looks: Dress Number 2 by itself, a Vest, and a Jacket

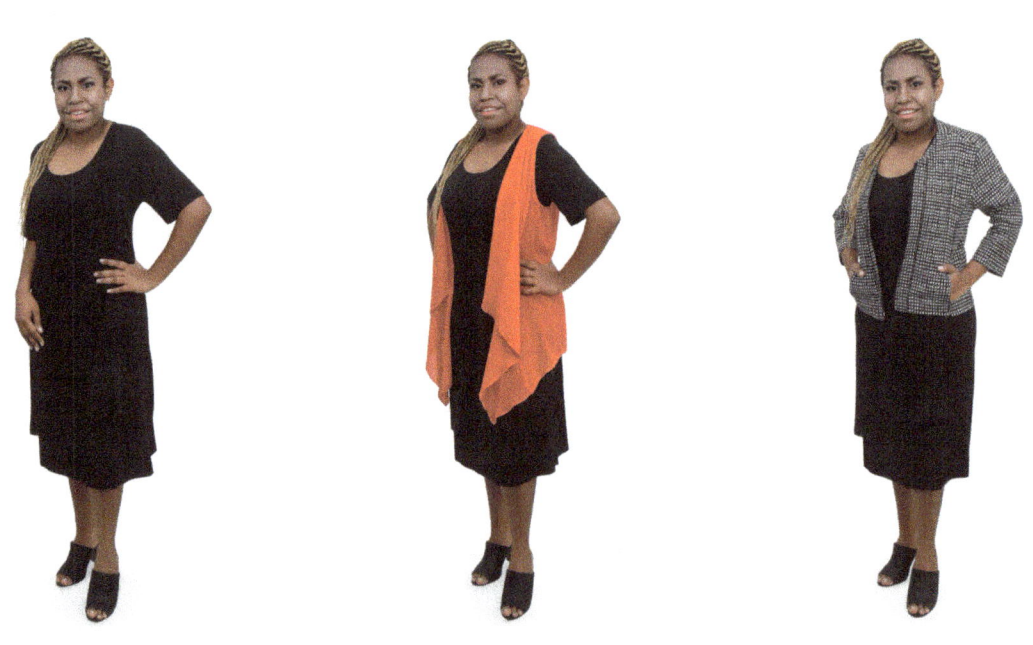

Examples of Mix-and-Match Wardrobes

There are a lot of mix-and-match wardrobe ideas out there, and on the following pages are a few examples for women working/living in different scenarios. The selections will help you come to a decision quicker on what to wear when you are standing in front of your wardrobe.

Also bear in mind that not all women are fortunate to have the example of the mix-and-match wardrobe at once. That is why you must build your perfect mix-and-match wardrobe over time or as your budget allows. When you are caring for your clothes through the correct washing and drying techniques, it can last for many years. You will also reach your full mix-and-match wardrobe sooner if you do not have to replace garments all the time. I have proven results where some of my stylish clothes have lasted for ten years. At the end of this book, I will elaborate more on how to care for your clothes the right way.

Bras and underwear need replacing more regularly because they contain elastic. When elastic is stretching for long times, it gets worn out and does not return to its original form. I have had quality bras that lasted me three to four years. However, I have cared for them very well and did not wear the same one every day. I have rotated each on a six-day schedule. A bra and shapewear have a job to do, and once it is deformed and has lost its shape, it cannot perform its job properly and will also become uncomfortable to wear. Our underwear dictates how our clothes display on us. Therefore, your underwear can make or break how your outfit appears. Another important thing to remember is to never wear underwear for more than a day without washing them. You can get away with wearing a bra for two days, not consecutive, before washing it; but only in winter or cold climates.

How one kills a bra quicker:

- not giving it enough resting time by wearing it every day (solution: have more bras and rotate them; one for every day of the week is ideal).
- buying the cheapest bras, which normally do not last long.
- wrong washing and drying techniques.
- bra cups being squished (keep it up at all times even when placing in a drawer).
- washing by machine and not by hand (bras are delicate garments and need to be hand-washed delicately).

Women in a Corporate Job and Relaxing at Home

Seventy-five per cent of your wardrobe should look like this:

- two work trousers with zippers (black, navy, brown, grey, deep beige)
- three pencil skirts (black, navy, brown, grey, deep beige)
- two comfortable pull-up trousers
- two dresses (one colourful and one in one colour)
- one corporate long-sleeved jacket (choose a corporate colour fitting your job)
- two corporate shirts (white or the colour fitting your job)
- one evening dress (in a style that can look different each time by adding a jacket or evening shawl)
- two good-fitting and comfortable jeans (black or denim)
- two shorts or long shorts or three-quarter-length pants
- two T-shirts
- two sets of tracksuits
- seven underwear (mixture of briefs, bikinis, G-strings, etc.)
- two shapewear panties
- seven bras (to last a six-day washing cycle)
- one sports bra
- two pairs of comfortable work or professional shoes
- one pair of trainers or runners
- one pair of boots
- one pair of comfortable flat shoes

Twenty-five per cent of your wardrobe should look something like this: *

- two fashionable long-sleeved jackets (update when out of fashion)
- two short- or three-quarter-sleeved fashionable jackets
- three fashionable long or short-sleeveless vests
- seven colourful and fashionable long- and short-sleeved shirts
- two pairs of fashionable thongs or slip-ons
- one pair of high heels (in a colour that will fit most of your formal/evening wear).

*Update fashionable outfits when out of fashion.

Stay-at-Home Moms and Homemakers

Seventy-five per cent of your wardrobe should look something like this:

- one formal trousers (black, navy, brown, grey, deep beige)
- two pencil skirts (black, navy, brown, grey, deep beige)
- two pull-up comfortable trousers
- two dresses (one colourful and one in one colour)
- one evening dress (in a style that can look different each time by adding a jacket or evening shawl)
- two good-fitting comfortable jeans (black, denim)
- two shorts or long shorts or three-quarter-length pants
- two sets of tracksuits
- two sweaters
- four T-shirts
- seven underwear (mixture of briefs, bikinis, G-strings, etc.)
- two shapewear panties
- seven bras (to last a six-day washing cycle)
- one sports bra
- two pairs of comfortable shoes
- one pair of trainers or runners
- one pair of boots
- one pair of comfortable flat shoes
- two pairs of fashionable thongs or slip-ons.

Twenty-five per cent of your wardrobe should look something like this: *

- one fashionable long-sleeved jacket
- two fashionable short- or three-quarter-sleeved jackets
- two fashionable long or short-sleeveless vests
- four colourful and fashionable long- and short-sleeved shirts
- one pair of comfortable high heels (in a colour that will fit most of your formal and evening wear).

*Update fashionable outfits when out of fashion.

Young Ladies Studying or Working Part-Time

Seventy-five per cent of your wardrobe should look something like this:

- one formal trousers (black, navy, brown)
- two comfortable skirts (pencil, knee length, or mini in black, navy blue, brown)
- two comfortable pull-up trousers
- one evening dress (in a style that can look different each time by adding a jacket or evening shawl)
- two good-fitting comfortable jeans (black or denim)
- two shorts or long shorts or three-quarter-length pants
- two sets of tracksuits
- two sweaters
- four T-shirts
- seven underwear (mixture of briefs, bikinis, G-strings, etc.)
- two shapewear panties
- seven bras (to last a six-day washing cycle)
- one sports bra
- one pair of trainers or runners
- one pair of boots
- one pair of comfortable flat shoes
- one pair of fashionable thongs or slip-ons.

Twenty-five per cent of your wardrobe should look something like this: *

- one fashionable long-sleeved jacket
- two dresses (one colourful and one in one colour)
- two fashionable long or short, sleeveless vests
- three colourful and fashionable long- and short-sleeved shirts
- one pair of comfortable high or short heels (a colour that will fit most of your formal and evening wear).

*Update fashionable outfits when out of fashion.

A Woman Working as a Tradesperson

Seventy-five per cent of your wardrobe should look something like this:

- six company shirts
- six company trousers
- one formal trousers
- two comfortable pull-up trousers
- two comfortable dresses
- two good-fitting comfortable jeans (black or denim)
- two shorts or long shorts or three-quarter-length pants
- two sets of tracksuits
- two sweaters
- four T-shirts
- nine underwear (mixture of briefs, bikinis, G-strings, hipsters, boy shorts)
- one shapewear panty
- five sports bras
- three comfortable bras
- eight pairs of work socks
- one good quality and comfortable work boots
- one pair of trainers or runners
- one pair of boots
- one pair of flat comfortable shoes
- one pair of fashionable thongs or slip-ons

It depends on how many company shirts and trousers your work supplies, but the ideal should be enough to last on a six-day washing cycle.

Twenty-five per cent of your wardrobe should look something like this: *

- one fashionable long-sleeved jacket
- one fashionable long or short sleeveless vest
- three colourful and fashionable long- and short-sleeved shirts
- two dresses or skirts or trousers (or a mix)
- one pair of comfortable high or short heels (in a colour that will fit most of your formal and evening wear)

*Update fashionable outfits when out of fashion.

Of course, you can go outside the suggestions and create your own 75-25 per cent wardrobe.

Fashion and Body Proportions

Fashion and Body Proportions

Not all the new fashion styles will automatically fit every woman; and for this reason we can say that fashion is only good if it fits you well. The smart way is to adapt the latest fashion/trend to your body shape and personality, rather than trying to alter your body and personality to accommodate each trend.

Do not become obsessed with your flaws, but instead consider your blessings. You do not have to be a woman who wears a jacket that comes down to her knees to cover a large bottom, or who refuses to smile for the fear of exposing crooked teeth.

Acting uncomfortable looks suspicious and attracts more attention; people will wonder what you are hiding. When you look at your reflection in the mirror, you most likely focus on all the bulges, blemishes, and wrinkles. All your fears will disappear once you learn to construct, and project, a complete look that emphasizes your beauty, great personality, and best features. People that you meet will instead see an attractive woman with a warm, and genuine personality.

Use the information in this book to dress your best for your body shape and personality, but the most important characteristic is to be happy. Happiness hides a lot of imperfections. Therefore, a happy and friendly personality will override any negativity and imperfection.

In the case where you are not feeling happy, you must try your utmost best to find out what it is that makes you feel unhappy, then work towards it to improve or even take the drastic step of removing it from your life. Explore and find out what will make you happy, and put a plan in motion to work on moving to a happier and more successful you.

Regularly read and watch motivational content or join a community group. Another fantastic way is to volunteer. Help people who are less fortunate than you; it gives you the sense of purpose and a fresh perspective on which blessings you need to be grateful for. There is no use in trying to be someone else, but be the best version you can be of yourself. That is when you are the happiest.

Body Posture

Good posture helps keep bones and joints in the correct alignment so that muscles are used properly to avoid the developing of an abnormal permanent position. Proper posture also reduces abnormal wear and tear on joint surfaces, which can lead to arthritis. It decreases the stress on the ligaments holding the joints of the spine together. Good posture and back support are essential for avoiding back and neck pain. It enhances proper breathing, ensuring oxygen and nutrients going to all the organs for optimal health and functioning.

Carole Jackson explained posture in fashion the best: Your posture dictates how good your clothes look on you. The most expensive and beautifully fitted garments cannot overcome the unflattering effect of a slouching body. The lines of your clothes will hang more gracefully if your shoulders are held upright and your tummy and bottom are tucked in. Stand straight with your weight distributed evenly on both feet. Imagine a string running from your chest bone to the ceiling, suspending you like a marionette. Now drop your shoulders and shake your head slightly from side to side. You should now be standing correctly. Regularly practise standing this way in front of a mirror, and walk while pulling up through your midriff, head held high and shoulders down. Swing your legs from the joint at the hip rather than the knee when you walk. This way of walking is smooth and elegant.

You can definitely change your body posture through focusing on how you walk and sit every day. The time frame on developing a beautiful and upright body posture depends on yourself and how badly you want it. Regular exercise, going to the gym, or working with a personal trainer can speed up the process. If you find it hard to correct your body posture on your own, it may be a wise decision to visit the chiropractor to see if there are easier ways.

Walking or sitting a certain way for years may have pulled muscles into wrong positions. Sometimes our muscles have lost its strength or shape because of bad posture. The vertebrae could also have moved slightly, that will need a chiropractor's help to correct. Through persevering every day, you will be able to change your posture and eventually reap all the benefits of it. Good posture not only helps our clothing appear more elegant on us but it also has numerous health benefits.

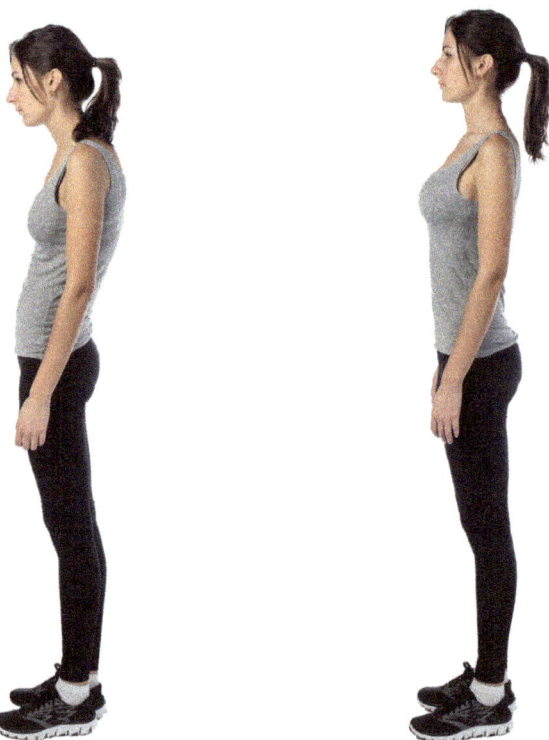

Example of a slouching body and good posture.

Body Proportions

Understanding your own body proportions will enable you to know how to use lines and colours to bring out your best features. Only a minority of women have the perfect body proportions and can wear almost anything. Further on, I'll explain more on how you can create the perfect proportioned body illusion through line design and colour. This is called optical illusion.

The perfect way to determine your body proportions as Carole Jackson advised in her book *Color Me Beautiful*:

- Stand bare feet against a door and ask someone to make tiny pencil marks or use a masking tape to indicate where each shoulder bone and hip bone is situated.
- Measure the difference between the marks. If your hips are more than 1 inch or 3 centimetres wider than your shoulders, or vice versa, you can take steps to give the illusion of a better proportion through optical illusion.
- Next, mark your height. Then mark your leg length at the point where your thigh joint 'breaks' from the hip.
- Now, measure both distances from the floor. The average leg length is half of your entire height. If your measurements reveal a discrepancy of more than 1 inch or 3 centimetres either way, you will want to use camouflage through line design and optical illusion.
- Slightly long legs are often an advantage because our eyes find it pleasing when the lower half of the body appears longer than the top half. That is why models are made to appear that they have longer legs. They are creating an optical illusion to make the legs appear longer.
- Mark the door now at your waist and then your armpit. The well-positioned waist falls in the middle between your armpit and the leg break, and a variation of more than an inch or three centimetres define you as either high-waisted or low-waisted.
- Lastly, look at the size of your head in relation to your body. A small head gives the illusion of height, while a large head shortens. If your head seems too small or too large, adjust your hairstyle, making it either closer to your face to compensate for a large head or fuller for a small one.

The Three Body Types

There are three general categories of female body types: the ectomorph, mesomorph, and endomorph. In fact, most people can have a combination of two body types. The combinations can be either mesomorph/endomorph or ectomorph/mesomorph. It is also not uncommon to find a pure mesomorph gaining weight like an endomorph.

It's important to note that it is extremely rare for an individual to show 100 per cent of the characteristics for their body type. We all display some characteristics from each body type; however, one type will generally dominate. The dominant type of characteristics determines the actual body type that we are assigned to.

Ectomorph

· thin build · narrow hips and clavicles · small wrist and ankles · long limbs · stringy muscle bellies · flat chest · fast metabolism · difficulty gaining weight · difficulty gaining muscle

Mesomorph

· athletic build · wide shoulders · seems to burn fat quickly · thinner joints · well-defined muscles · narrow waist · gains muscle easily · low body fat

Endomorph

· soft and round body · larger frame · thick ribcage · wide and thicker joints · difficulty losing weight · hips are as wide as or wider than clavicles · gains muscle and fat easy

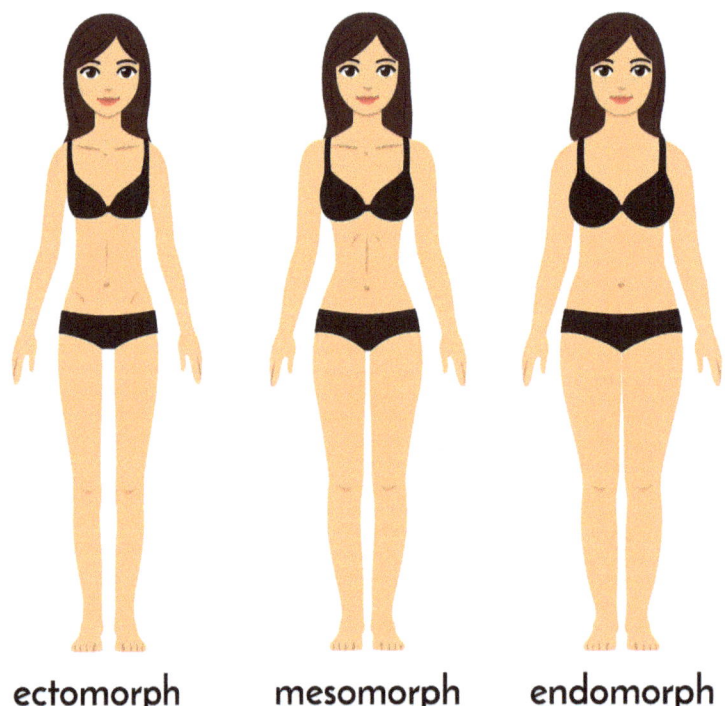

ectomorph   mesomorph   endomorph

An *ectomorph* is a typical slim figure. Ectomorphs have a light build with small joints and lean muscle. Usually, they have long thin limbs with stringy muscles. Shoulders tend to be thin with little width. The lean body shape, the slim petite, or the very slim hourglass body shapes fall into this category. This body type finds it hard to build muscle and has a small bust.

A *mesomorph* has a large bone structure, large muscles, and a naturally athletic physique. Mesomorphs find it quite easy to gain and lose weight. They are naturally strong. The inverted triangle, hourglass, slimmer rectangle, or stronger petite body shapes fall into this category.

The e*ndomorph* body type is solid and generally soft. Endomorphs gain fat very easily and are usually of a shorter build with thick arms and legs. Muscles are strong, especially the upper legs. The round, pear, larger rectangle, or plus-size body shapes normally fall into this category. The overweight petite body shape can also be an endomorph.

The Scale of Body Shapes and Sizes

The scale of a garment print should be compatible with the wearer's body shape and size. A petite body shape would be intimidated by too large bold prints as small prints would on a larger body shape.

How to do a quick assessment of your body scale without measuring:

- Wrap your middle finger and thumb around the wrist of your dominant hand. Right-handed women will wrap their right hand and left-handed the left hand.
- When fingers easily touch or overlap your wrist, you are small scale.
- When your fingers just touch, you are medium scale.
- When your fingers are 1 centimetre (about 0.5 inch) or more apart, you are large scale.

Small Print   **Medium Print**   **Large Print**

The following assessments will give a more realistic scale, as they take into account your height, weight, and bone structure.

Small Scale

You have a small body scale if you have the following measurements:

- wrist measurement of less than 14 centimetres (5.5 inches).
- a height of less than 161 centimetres (5 feet 4.5 inches).
- weight either slightly under or slightly over what's recommended for your height and bone structure.

Medium Scale

You have a medium body scale if you have the following measurements:

- wrist measurement of 14 centimetres to 16.5 centimetres (5.5 inches to 7.5 inches).
- height at or above 161 centimetres to 170 centimetres (5 feet 4.5 inches to 5 feet 7 inches).
- weight that is either within normal range or moderately overweight for your height and bone structure.

Large Scale

You are a large body scale if you have the following measurements:

- wrist measurement of larger than 16.5 centimetres (7.5 inches).
- height above 170 centimetres (5 feet 7 inches).
- weight that is normal or moderately overweight for your height and bone structure.

When the patterns are small and wider apart with a one-tone colour in between, it will have the same effect as large print, because the large gaps in between the small patterns will give the illusion of being large.

The Eight Different Body Shapes

We all have a vague idea of what category we think our body shape may fit into. The subject on body shapes is not common knowledge. In this section, you'll learn how to differentiate between the eight body shapes, and to discover yours. Knowing your body shape will assist you to determine which clothing styles will suit your figure best and how you can hide the less-flattering features.

During our lifetime, we can easily be two to three different body shapes. It is not uncommon for a woman to be a lean body shape when she is young and then change to a rectangle- or round body shape as she gets older. This section is dedicated to make you feel better about yourself through knowing the correct styling techniques. Let's face it, we do not all look like a bikini model. Staying fit and in shape is a full-time job, and not all of us have the luxury to stay at home, let alone, make time every day to stay fit.

An obsession with our body image is unhealthy and can lead to social isolation, eating disorders, and even depression. Do not let your body image get in the way of a happy and successful life. Endeavour to involve movement in your every day. If you sit on the couch all day long, you will not maintain your body weight and for sure not lose the extra kilograms that you wish to lose in order to feel healthier and happier. When you keep your weight consistently within a variation of 2-3 kilograms from your normal weight and not gain too much weight, you'll gain around 500 grams to 1 kilogram (1-2 pounds) per year on average, without a regular exercise or movement program.

Work extra movement into your daily routine through parking as far as you can from the shops, taking the stairs rather than the escalators or elevators, doing your own housecleaning, washing the floors by hand on your knees on a knee cushion or while crouching if you are able to without hurting yourself, washing your house's windows inside and out, hanging up your washing on washing lines that allow you to stretch a bit, washing your car, doing some gardening. Who needs to go to the gym if you can get free exercise through your daily routine! Be careful if you are not used to these kinds of jobs. Start slowly and always warm up first.

A Quick Characteristics Guide

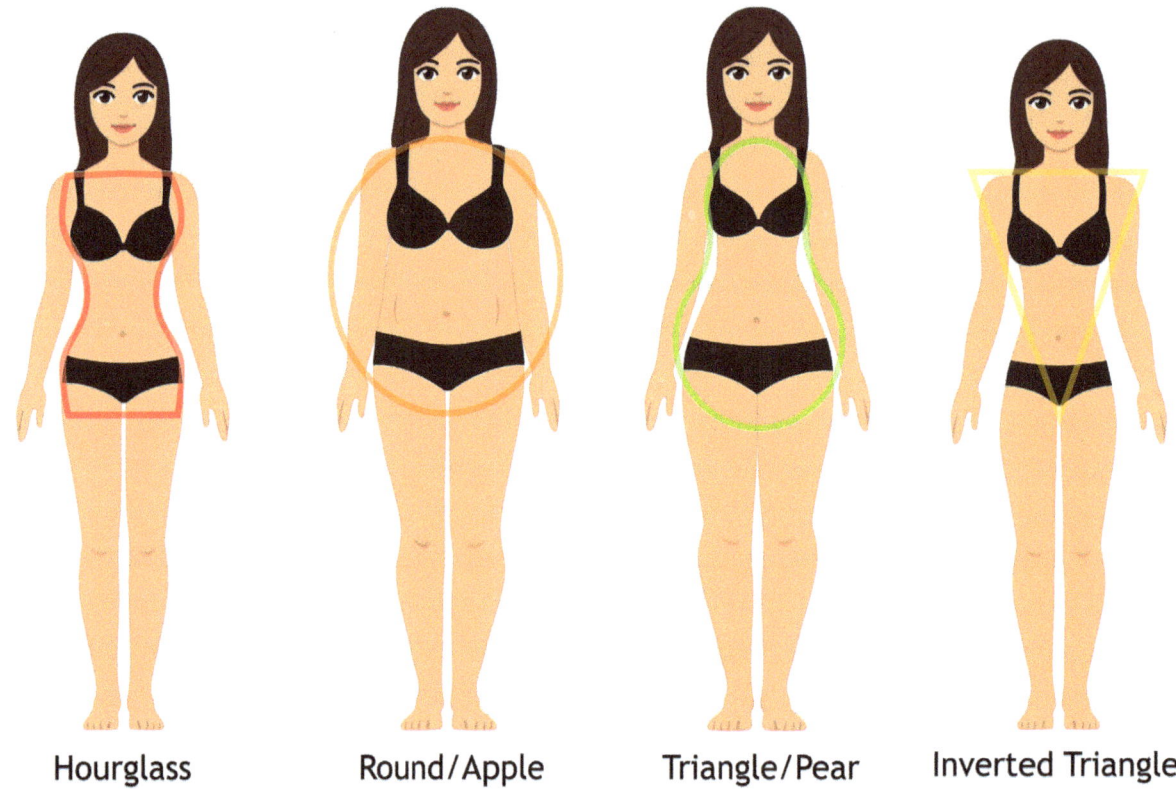

Hourglass   Round/Apple   Triangle/Pear   Inverted Triangle

Hourglass	**Round/Apple**
• has softly rounded curves. • shoulders and hips in equal proportion. • small waist defined as an hourglass. • aligned bust-line and hips. • the most flattering figure to the eye.	• soft figure and round from the bust to the hips. • shoulders and hips in proportion, larger waistline/tummy. • slimmer thighs, great legs. • difficulty in defining the waist.
Triangle/Pear	**Inverted Triangle**
• illusion of looking shorter because of the wide hips and bottom. • shoulders and waist smaller than the hips and bottom. • the sexiest figure to most men, if not overweight. • elegant neck, slim arms, and shoulders.	• the swimmer figure with athletic shoulders and no or little bust-line. • can also be a heart figure recognized by large breasts. • the upper arms appear wider than the shoulders. • small waist and bottom, great legs.

for the Eight Different Body Shapes

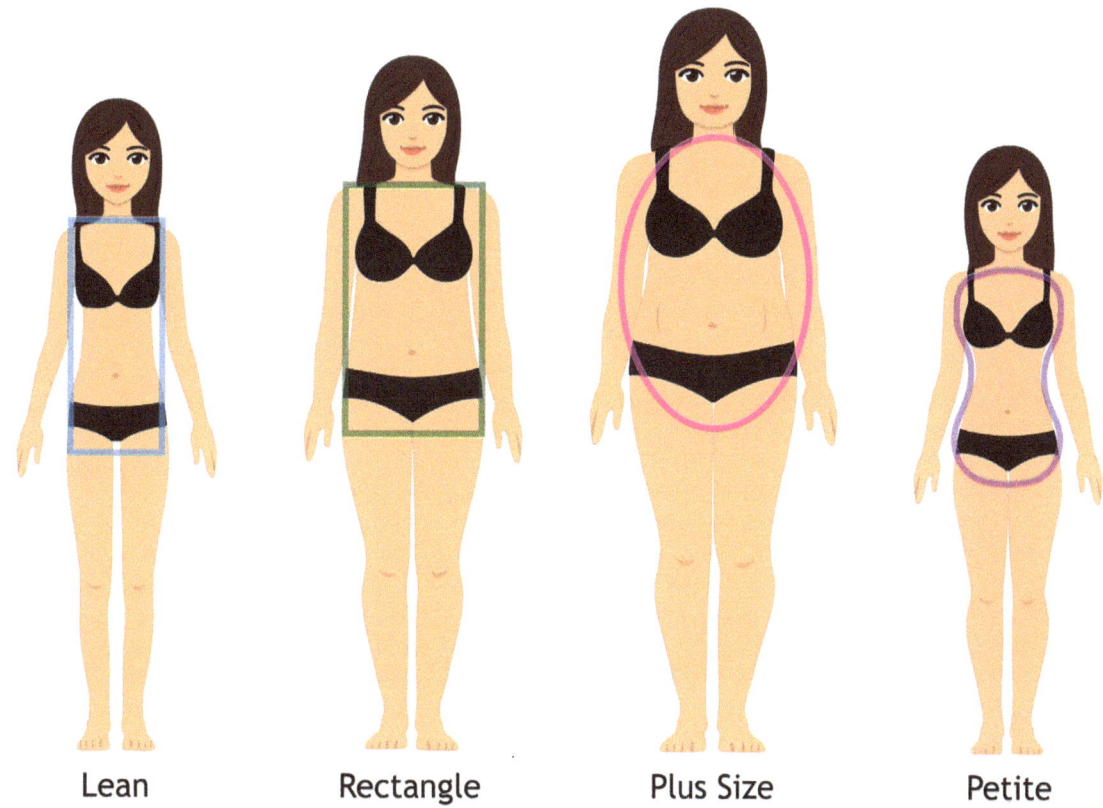

Lean	Rectangle
• square or rectangle figure that may or may not have a waist. • shoulders, hips, and waist all in proportion and quite lean. • silhouette with straight lines. • flat chest, small bust, and flat bottom.	• bust and hips approximately of the same width. • shoulders in proportion to the waist and hips, and squared. • very little waist definition, good legs. • gained weight distributed evenly.
Plus Size	**Petite**
• tall in height or bigger in size (can be both). • bigger than a size 16. • very curvy and carries extra weight. • large hips and bottom. • great bust-line.	• short in height, generally below 158 centimetres. • short through the torso and short legs. • can be any of the following body shapes: hourglass, rectangle, pear/triangle, inverted triangle, round/apple or lean figure.

Reasons Why Our Body Shape Changes as We Get Older

Hormones

As menopause approaches in a woman's life, three hormones, (oestrogen, progesterone, and testosterone) gradually decline. Therefore, fat in the body begins to deposit around the belly and inside the belly as well as around the hips and thighs.

Lack of Exercise

A lot of women become less active because life gets in the way. Having children and bringing them up is a full-time job and all the other chores that come from being a wife and mother. Other reasons for slowing down in activity can range from having a disability, or medical condition, or retiring from work and not being as active any more. The biggest problem is that being more sedentary means having less muscle mass, and muscle mass is necessary for effective calorie burning.

Overeating

Doing slight changes to our diet will assist us in not consuming too much calories. Cut out fizzy drinks and diet sodas. People are under the misconception that they will not gain weight when they drink diet sodas. These are loaded with artificial sweeteners, which have been shown to cause weight gain. In 2016 studies done by the University of Sydney in both animals and humans have suggested that consuming artificial sweeteners can make you feel hungry and actually eat more. For more information on this subject, google 'why artificial sweeteners can increase appetite', The University of Sydney.

Osteoporosis

Osteoporosis comes with age and can cause rounding in the spine and shoulders. It does not have to be a problem if we take in enough calcium and keep up with an exercise program. Osteoporosis is a medical condition in which bones become brittle and fragile from loss of tissue, typically as a result of hormonal changes, or deficiency of calcium or vitamin D. Brittle bones become smaller and shorter. That is why a lot of older people will look shorter and their body shape will take on another shape as they get older.

Gravity

As we age, our bodies also naturally begin to sag in places. Breasts often drop, and a belly can pull down if a person is overweight. This is another reason for the change in body shape.

Style Personalities

Our personality and lifestyle play a major part in our personal style. Clothes we wear generally reflect our personality. The job that we are in, also dictates our personal dress style. Obviously, a tradeswoman or archaeologist is not going to dress in corporate clothes and high heels when she goes to work, which can be a lot of times out there in the field. How uncomfortable would that be? On the other hand, it is not appropriate for a lawyer to represent a case in the court in her tracksuit.

Style personality types can be divided into five styles, and many of us can be a combination of two.

1. *Natural* Personality

- The natural's look is relaxed with ease of movement.
- They feel comfortable in jeans, trousers, shorts, and simple tops.
- They require easy caring for, practical, hard-wearing, and non-fussy clothes.
- They wear little make-up and/or no jewellery.
- When they wear classic clothes to work, they take them off as soon as they get home and swap it for more comfortable clothes.

2. *Contemporary* Personality

- The contemporary type has to have the latest fashion.
- They are very aware of fashion trends and will buy the latest garments as soon as they are released on the market. Just as the tech savvy guy will stand in a line for hours to get their hands on the latest iPhone model, so will the contemporary personality for clothes.
- The fashionable look is easy to achieve; just add the current season's accessories or colour as part of your outfit.

3. *Classic* Personality

- The classic type always looks smart, neat, and tidy. They avoid fabrics that crease easily.
- They like a formal look even when dressed casually.
- When they wear jeans, it will be washed and ironed.
- Classics enjoy shopping for clothes and look for good quality, clean lines, and not high fashion.
- They will wear a small amount of make-up, small jewellery, including pearls.
- Shoes will always be clean and polished.

4. *Creative* Personality

- Creative types have an artistic flair.
- They alter their clothes to make their appearance unique and individualistic.
- They love interesting patterns, textures, colours, and scarves.
- They accessorize their outfits with creative jewellery, like large earrings and necklaces which are often in wood or ceramics or handmade pieces.
- They will spend hours looking for interesting items, and they enjoy shopping in unusual shops and markets.

5. *Dramatic* Personality

- They love to shop and normally forget practicality and budget.
- They need high fashion, often called 'street fashion'.
- They are likely to love hats and sunglasses on cloudy days, eye-catching jewellery, and full make-up.
- They need to stand out in a crowd and often belong to peer groups who like wearing the same type of dramatic clothing and shoes with enormous platforms.

Line-, Symmetrical-, Asymmetrical Designs And Creating Optical Illusion with Line Design

Line Design

Clothes can reveal or disguise our natural body contour. Clothing lines and shapes can be used to emphasize a person's good features and hide or minimize the less attractive ones.

The immediate effect of lines is as follows: With horizontal lines, we create width, and with vertical lines, we create height and a slimming effect. Diagonal lines draw attention and create points of interest as they intersect with other lines. It also creates a slight effect of height and slimming.

Vertical Lines

- create height.
- give the illusion of more body height and less width.
- draw attention away from the outlines of the body and create illusion of slenderness.

Horizontal Lines

- create width.
- balance another area, for example, the pear body shape's top and bottom.
- attract attention to body parts.
- tend to broaden and shorten a figure.

Diagonal Lines

- create more height than a horizontal lines.
- creating a slight slimming effect.
- diagonal lines are attention grabbing and create points of interest.

Line design in a garment can be created as follows:

- printed patterns in the fabric.
- fabric weaving texture.
- accessories (for example, a belt and scarfs).
- outline of the garment and the style lines within, that divide the garment. (for example, yokes, wide waistbands, extended shoulders, necklines, pressed pleats, tucks, buttoned front closures, V-necklines, and visible seams).

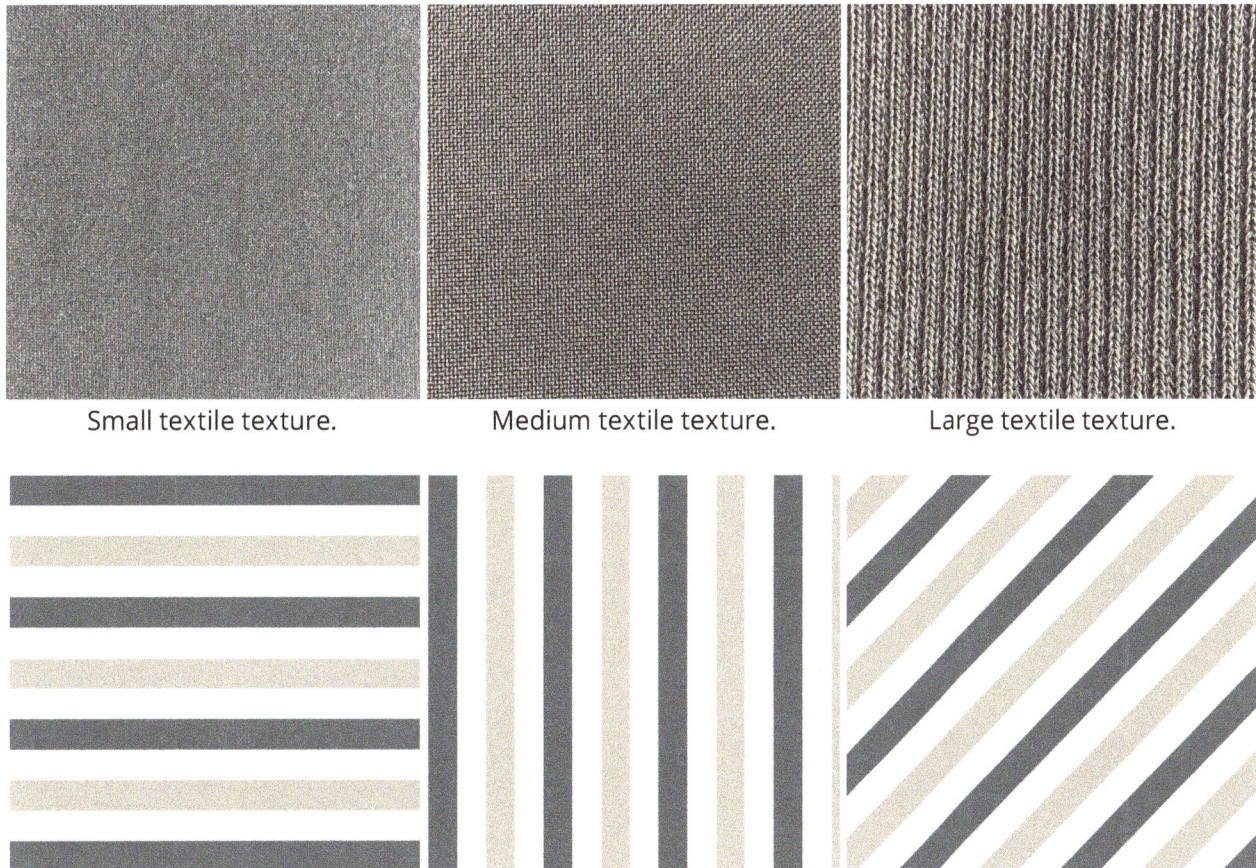

Symmetrical and Asymmetrical Designs

Asymmetric design is an attention-grabbing technique that is interesting and thought-provoking. Even the slightest bit of asymmetry can throw off the balance in a design. Asymmetrical hemlines are very feminine and attractive. Petite women must avoid wearing mid-calf length (halfway between the knee and the ankle), and asymmetrical handkerchief styles or jagged hemlines, as these lines can make her look even smaller and shorter. Asymmetric elements in garments can appear in hemlines, necklines, sleeves, shoulders, gathers, layers, slits, wraps, prints, patterns, etc.

Symmetrical

The space within a garment is divided into equal parts. Both sides of the axis look the same and are balanced.

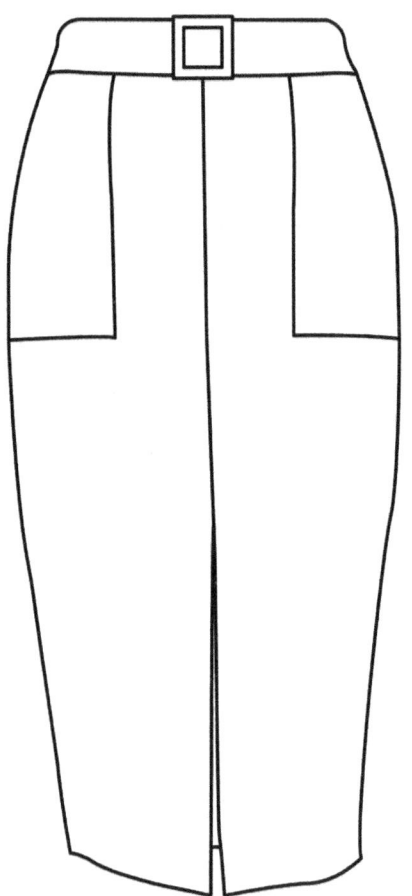

Asymmetrical

The space within a garment is divided unequally. The two sides of the axis look different and are not balanced.

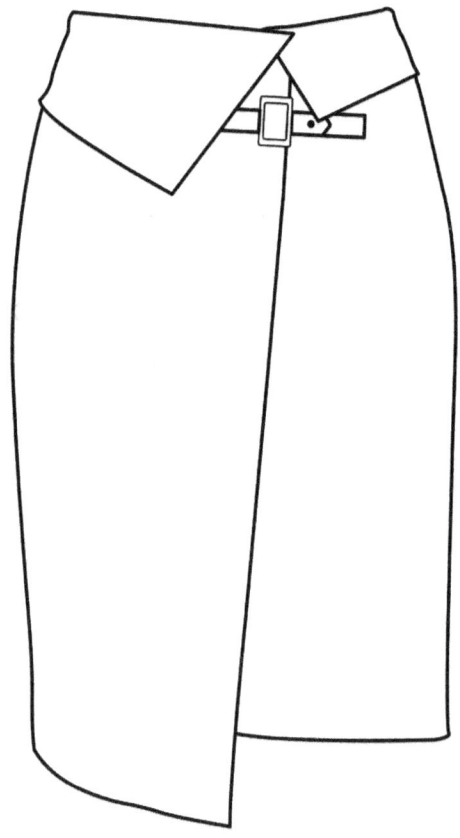

Symmetrical	**Asymmetrical**
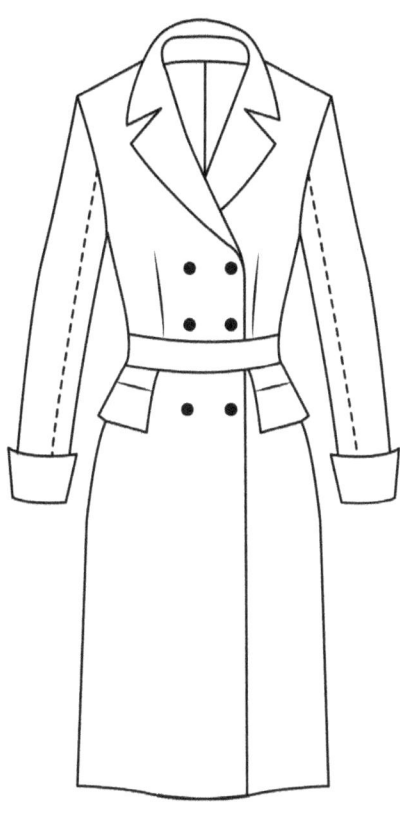	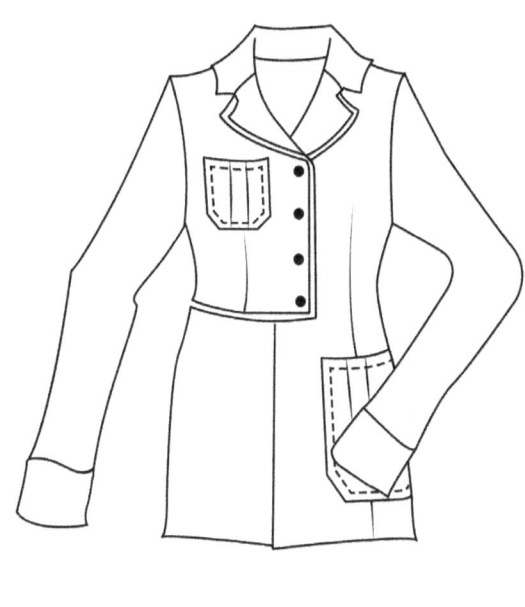
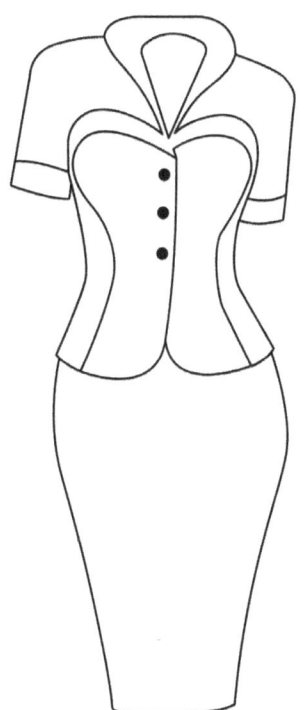	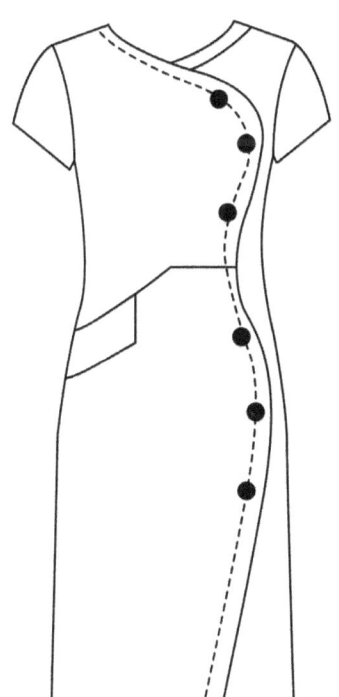

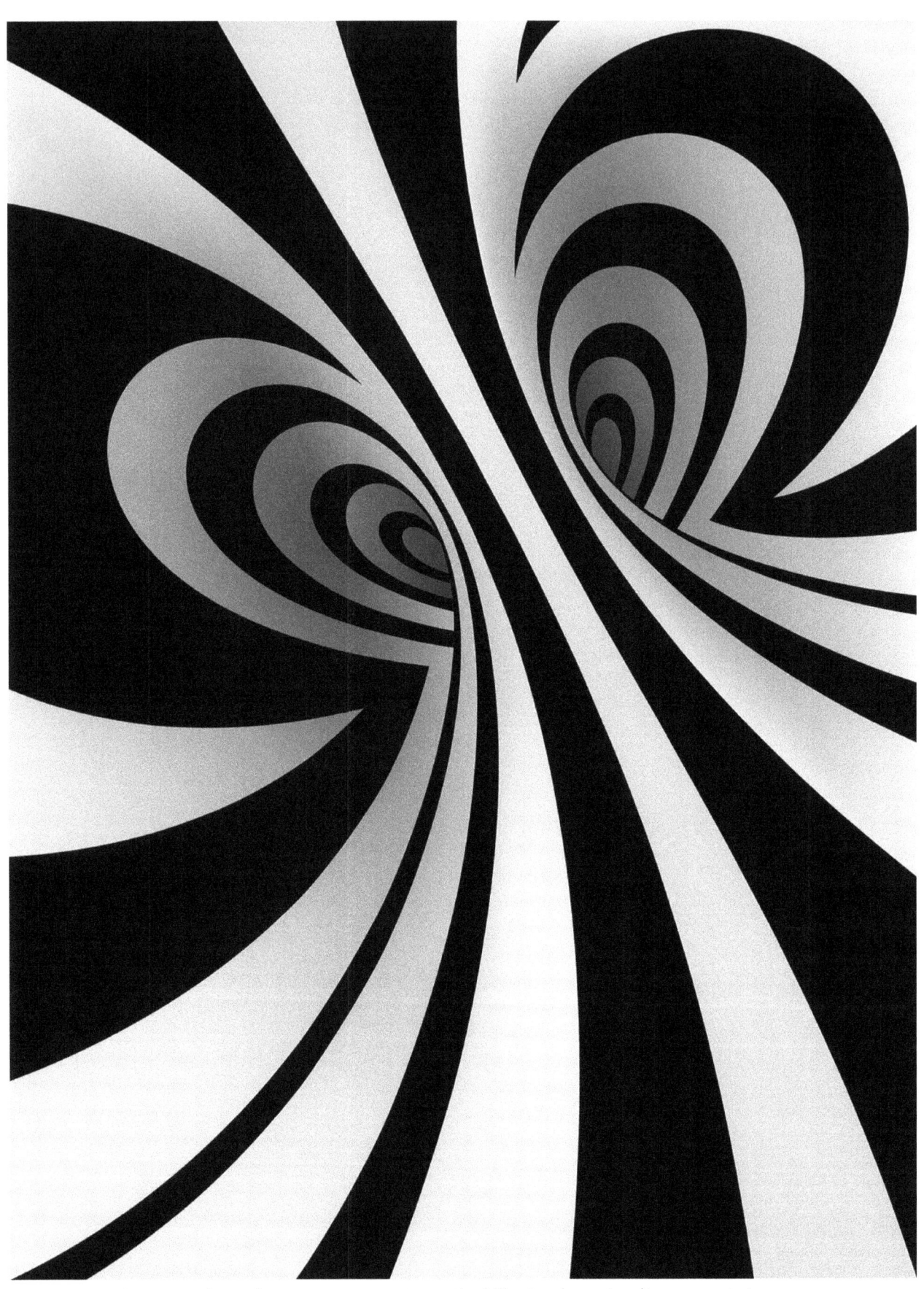
An example on how you can create optical illusion by using lines a certain way.

Creating Optical Illusion with Line Design

With line design, one can create an optical illusion of how we want things to look rather than how it looks in reality. It is a brilliant way to enhance the areas of our body that we want to show off, while, at the same time, minimize or hide the parts that we are conscious of.

This is the definition of *optical illusion* in the dictionary: A perception, as of visual stimuli (optical illusion) that represents what is perceived in a way different from the way it is in reality.

We basically trick the eye with clever ways of defining our waistline, creating a fuller bust area, minimizing the hips, appearing shorter or taller.

Different Features That Can Be Used to Create an Optical Illusion

- *Horizontal lines* - create width.
- *Waistbands* - balance areas.
- *Vertical lines* - create height and a slimming effect.
- *Diagonal lines* - create a slight slimming effect and height.
- *Colour(s)* - that are darker make areas appear smaller, and colours that are light or bright make areas appear larger.
- *Outlines of a garment* - create horizontal-, vertical-, and diagonal lines.
- *Necklines* - balance areas and can also be used to complement your face shape and chest area.
- *Pleats in a garment* - create horizontal-, vertical-, and diagonal lines. Pleats create a fuller effect.
- *Tucks and visible seams* - create horizontal-, vertical-, and diagonal lines.
- *Buttoned front closures* - create horizontal-, vertical-, and diagonal lines.

Vertical Lines

The closer the lines are spaced together, the slimmer you will look. Therefore, thinner lines are more slimming than wider lines.

Horizontal Lines

Horizontal lines will make you appear wider in the body part or area it is used.

These lines can also be used to balance an area. For example, women with wider hips than chest or breasts can wear horizontal lines in the upper body garments which help to make it appear smaller.

Horizontal lines used in the middle of the body figure make it appear shorter. Therefore, short women need to take care not to wear wide horizontal lines across their middle such as a belt, band, or scarf.

Diagonal Lines

Diagonal lines have a slight slimming effect, which is dependent on the degree of the angle.

The closer the lines are to vertical lines, the more slimming it is to the body figure, and in this case, they create height.

The closer the diagonal lines are to horizontal lines, the less slimming they are and may even make certain areas appear wider.

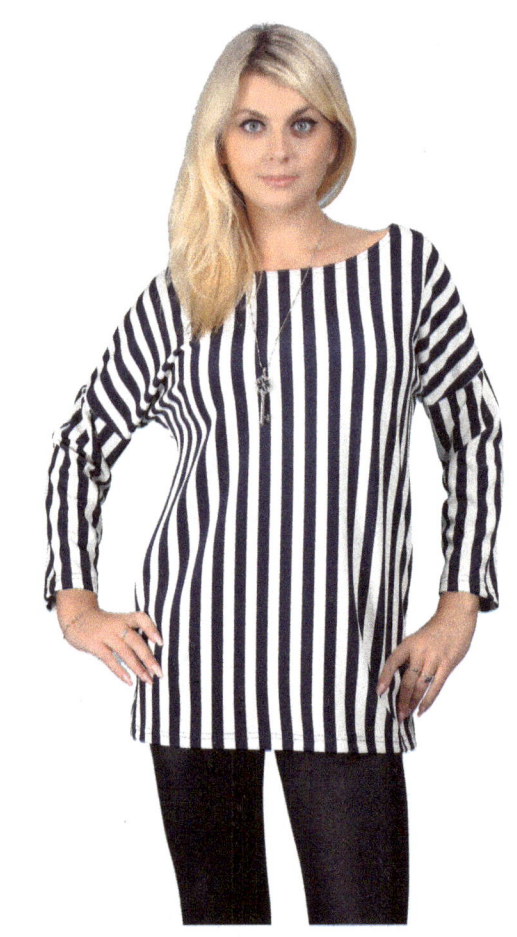

Vertical lines have a slimming effect and create height. Closer lines are more slimming.

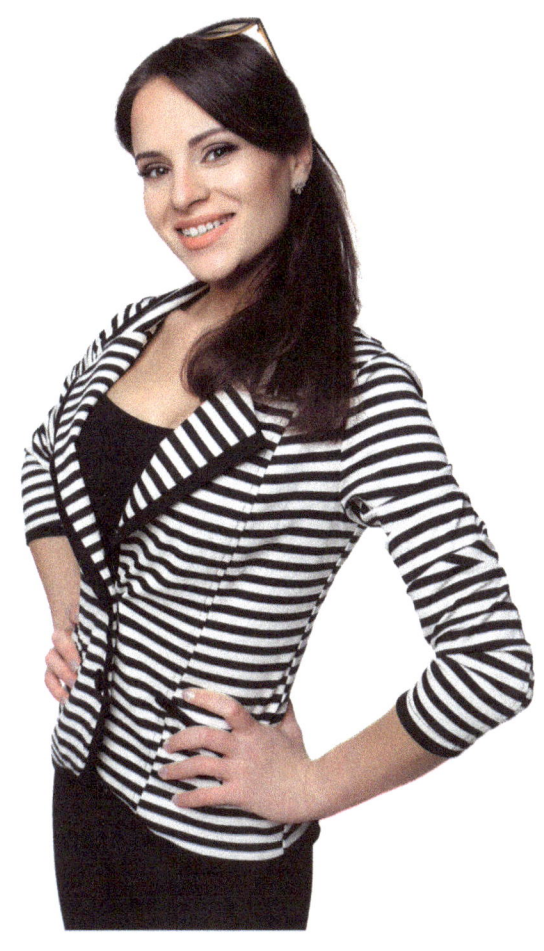 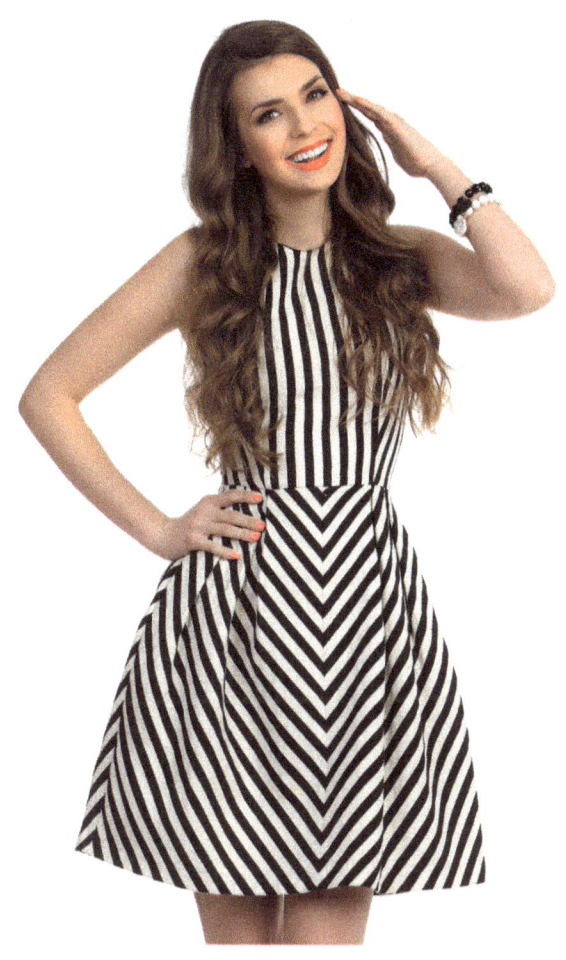

Horizontal lines create width from side to side, will enlarge any area, and can be used to balance areas.

Diagonal lines have a slight slimming effect and create height. Closer diagonal lines are more slimming.

The Best Necklines for Each Face Shape and Body Shape

Necklines and Face Shapes

Avoid wearing a neckline shape that's the same as your face shape if you do not want to draw attention to your face shape. For example, when you have a broad jawline, avoid a square neckline, a neckline that's straight across, or a boat neckline that is more straight and close to the face.

Here are a few tips:

- When you have a round face shape, do not wear a garment that has a round neckline.
- When you have a square or rectangle face shape, avoid a square neckline.
- The diamond, triangle, and heart face shapes must avoid triangular necklines, such as the V-neckline or sweet heart neckline because it will attract attention to the pointy chin and jawline.
- Wear high necklines for long to medium necks.
- Low necklines look better with short to medium necks.

The Different Face Shapes

Look at the following face shapes to determine yours. After this section, you will be able to discover which necklines and eyeglasses will fit with your face shape the best to complement your facial features.

There are nine different women face shapes:

Oval Face Shape

- Forehead and the jawline are approximately the same width.
- Chin is round in shape with no hard lines.
- Jawline has a slight roundness to it.
- Forehead is slightly broader than the jaw.
- The face is widest at the cheekbones.

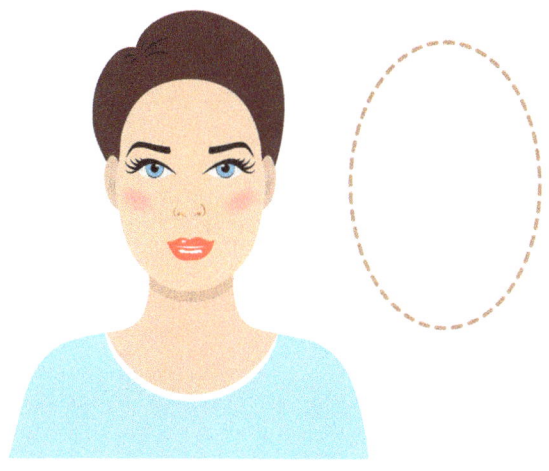

Oblong Face Shape

- Face is longer than it is wider and has a narrow width.
- Forehead and jawline appear similar in width.
- Cheeks and the sides of the face are straight.
- Forehead is tall and wide; it may be round at the hairline.
- Face is widest at the forehead, with a pointed chin.

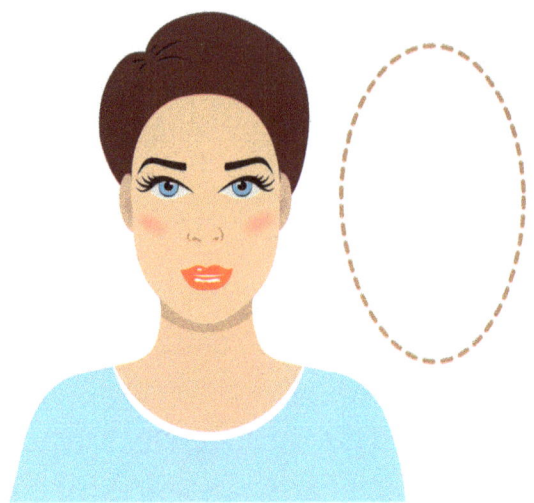

Diamond Face Shape

- Face is longer than it is wider.
- Forehead and jawline are a similar width in appearance, and forehead is narrow.
- Cheekbones are high and pointed.
- Jawline is long, and narrow and tapers into a point.
- Chin is noticeably pointed.

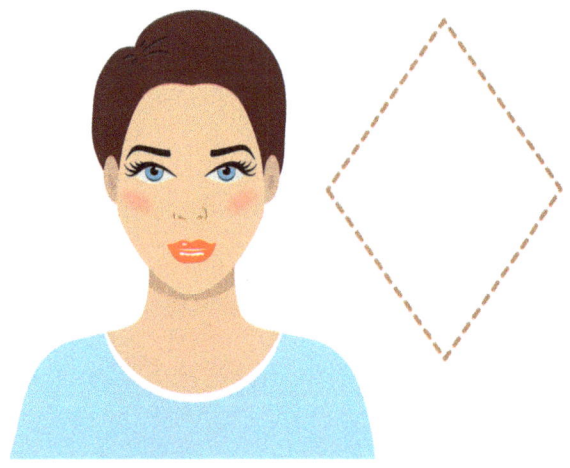

Rectangle Face Shape

- Face is longer than it is wider.
- Forehead and jawline are a similar width in appearance.
- Forehead is broad and most likely straight around the hairline.
- Cheeks and the sides of the face are straight.
- Chin is noticeably square and/or flat.

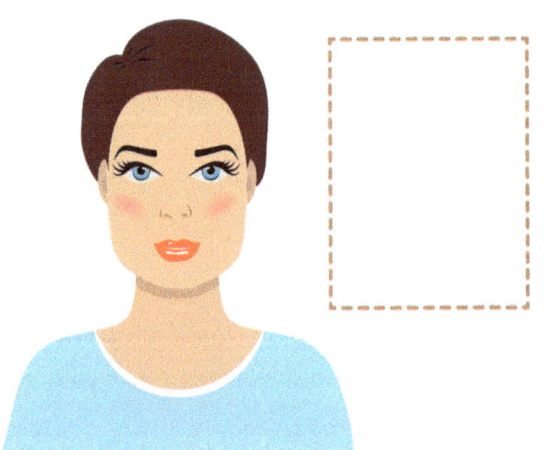

Square Face Shape

- Face is equal in length and width.
- Forehead and jawline are a similar width and most likely straight around the hairline.
- Jawline is strong, broad, and obviously square in appearance.
- Cheeks and the sides of the face are straight.
- Face is widest at the cheekbones.
- Chin is noticeably square and/or flat.

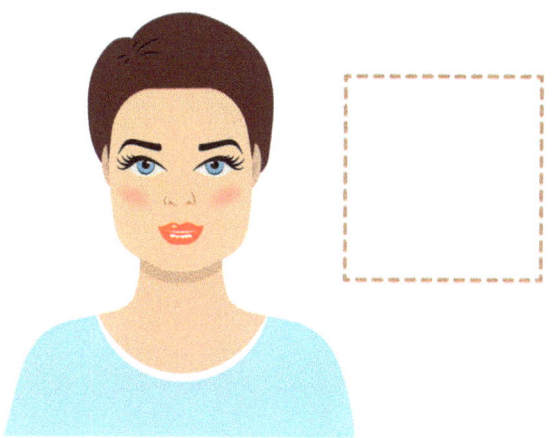

Heart Face Shape

- Face is longer than it is wider.
- Cheek line and the sides of the face taper into the jawline.
- Forehead is wide and round at the hairline.
- Face is widest at the forehead, and the cheekbones are wide and noticeable.
- Chin is noticeably pointed.

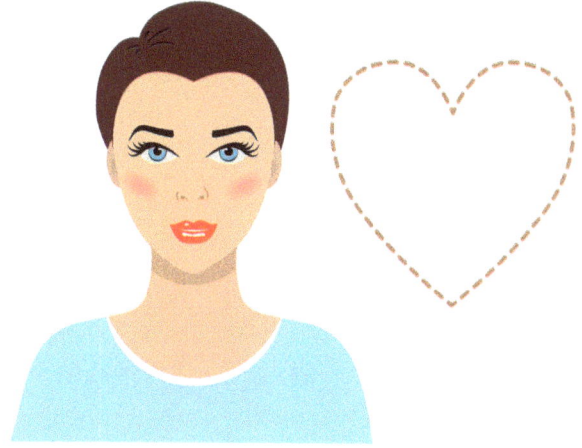

Triangle Face Shape

- Face is longer than it is wider.
- Jawline is wider than the forehead.
- Cheekbones are straight and taper from the jaw to the forehead.
- Face is widest at the jawline.
- Forehead is narrow.
- Chin is square and/or flat in shape.

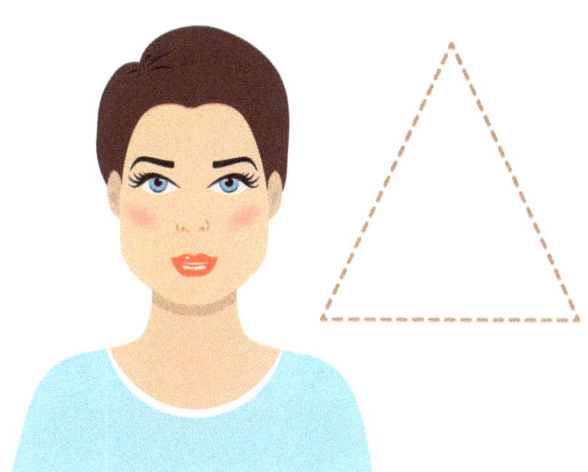

Inverted Triangle Face Shape

- Face is longer than it is wide.
- Face is widest at the forehead and almost straight at hairline.
- Cheekbones are wide and noticeable.
- Cheek line and the sides of the face taper into the jawline.
- Chin is noticeably pointed.

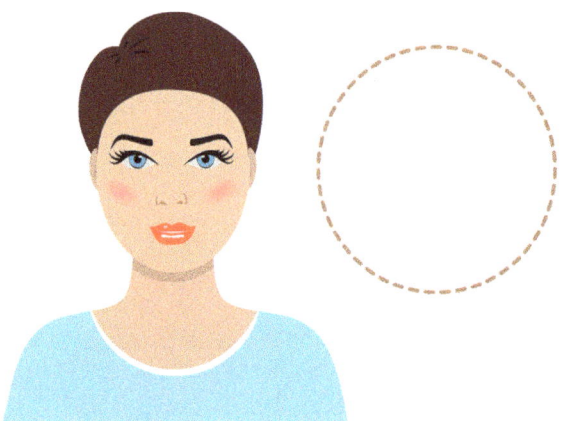

Round Face Shape

- Forehead and jawline are approximately the same width.
- The chin is rounded in shape with no hard lines.
- The jawline has a slight roundness to it.
- The forehead is slightly broader than the jaw.
- The face is widest at the cheekbones.

The Different Garment Necklines

A neckline is the top edge of a garment that surrounds the neck, and depending on the shape of the neckline, it can be close to the face or further away. The top-line really matters because it draws attention to your face and bosom. It is so important that it can make or break your looks.

When choosing the right necklines to wear, you should firstly determine your body proportions and select necklines that flatter those proportions. Secondly, choose a neckline that will accentuate your facial features.

If used correctly, the neckline can have the following outcomes:

- attracts attention to the centre of the body and soften broad shoulders.
- creates a leaner, longer, and taller silhouette figure.
- can elongate short necks or make long necks appear shorter.
- counteracts wide hips.
- can soften broad and strong jawlines.
- flatters a body shape.
- emphasizes beautiful collarbone and shoulder area.
- creates interesting focal points and make a statement.
- can create a balanced look.
- has a slimming effect on the bosom.
- makes shoulders appear wider or narrower.
- helps to minimize a large bust, or add volume to a smaller chest.

V-Neckline

The V-neck gives a vertical impression to the outfit; this type of neckline can create a leaner, longer, and taller silhouette. It draws the eye upward to the face, enhances the neck, and elongates the body.

For women who have broad shoulders, thick torsos, or short necks, this neckline is recommended. But overall, depending on the cut of the neckline, whether you are petite, slim, or a plus size, the V-neck flatters almost every figure. For those with a large bust, watch the cut. A very high V can make a large bust look saggy, while a plunging V can be too revealing. The wide V balances out pear body shapes.

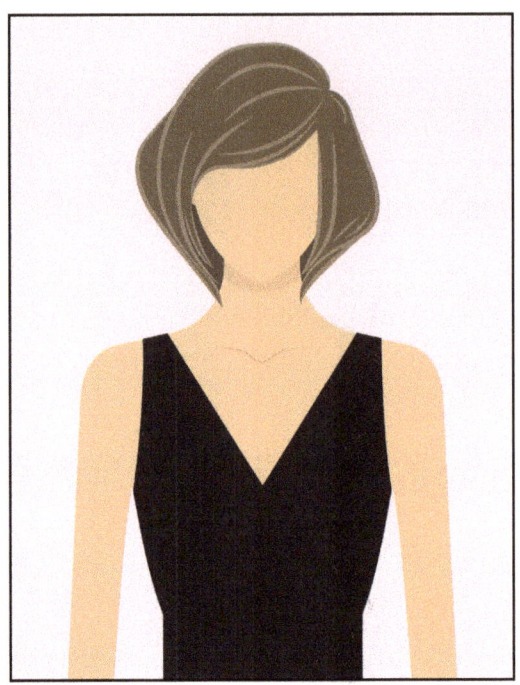

The V-neckline suits almost every body shape and size, but is best recommended for:

- those who have a large bust or have a little cleavage.
- full-figured women, as it gives a vertical illusion to the outfit.
- those with a short neck and broad shoulders, as it draws attention to the centre.
- those with wide, round, and square jaws, as it elongates the face shape.
- a good bra, will give maximum uplift and a great cleavage, and looks fabulous with the V-neckline.

Necklace Suggestions

Choose necklaces with contrasting shapes, such as round pendants or bead strands. Make sure it sits slightly above the V, or far below the V-neckline.

Square Neckline

Our collarbone and décolletage region is one of the most alluring parts of any woman. The square neckline is suitable for all body types. It helps to elongate a short neck and narrow shoulders.

If you are slim, petite, or small-chested, make sure you wear a fitted square neckline to give the illusion of curves to your bust-line. Don't forget to fill it out with a padded bra.

Women who have a square jawline must avoid a square neckline since it will draw attention to the squareness. All necklines that are not square or lined will work best for you.

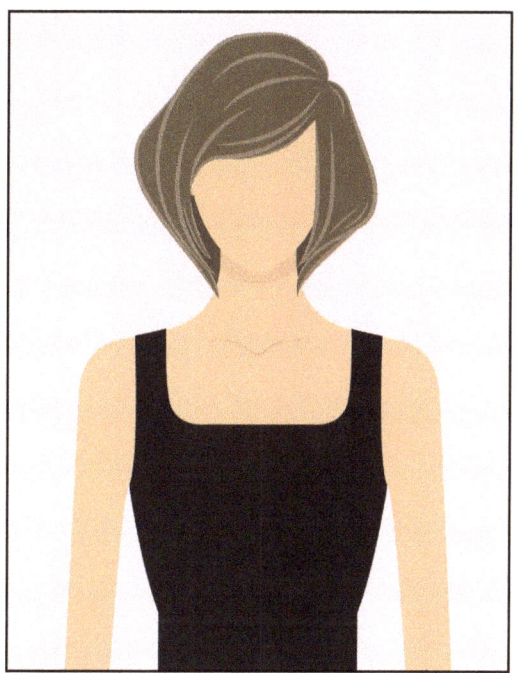

The square neckline suits almost every body shape and size except a body figure or face shape that is square. It is best recommended for:

- the round face shape to balance out the roundness.
- pear body shapes, as it helps to give the shoulders a broader look, therefore balancing the hips and shoulders.
- fat and/or short neck as it elongates your upper body.

Necklace Suggestions

Look for pendants with a round shape to harmonize the neckline's shape. Short layered chains, chokers, a dainty necklace, or a short chunky necklace are also good, as they create a structured round curve to complement and balance the square shape.

High Neckline or Turtle Neckline

High necklines have an extended tight-fitting high collar that tends to create volume in the neck area.

A true turtleneck that fits a couple of inches below the chin will chip away your height, making it best for those who want to offset a long neck or face.

Make sure to give room between the top of the turtleneck and your chin to avoid the floating head effect.

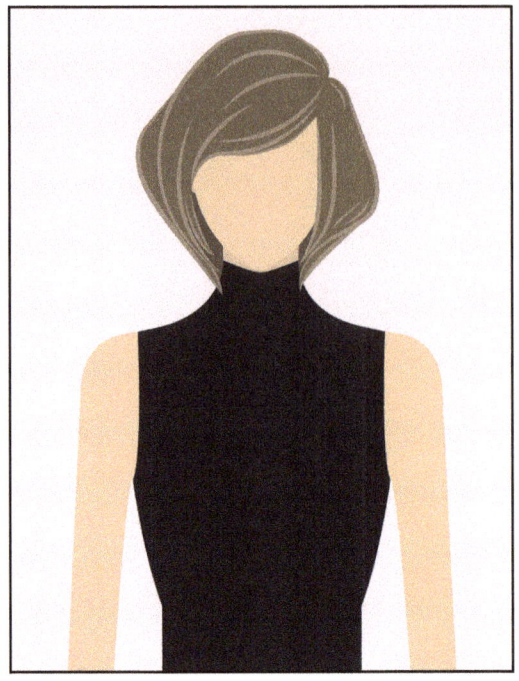

The high neckline or turtle neckline suits almost every body shape and size, but is best recommended for:

- small-chested women, as you will benefit more from high necklines, bulk or volume in the collar line area, is a great feature if your neck is relatively thin or long.
- those with a rectangle- or lean body shape; or those with narrow shoulders and faces, which take the most benefit from this neckline because this neckline draws the attention away from the squareness and narrowness.
- women with a long face shape or thin neck.

Necklace Suggestions

This neckline fits the most with long necklaces that are not too short and chunky, especially if you want to drag the attention away from a small or large bust area. Chunkier pieces look good and modern when worn over your turtleneck that ends halfway between the collarbone and bust-line.

Scoop Neckline

Generally, the scoop neckline can be worn by almost every body shape. This neckline displays the collarbone beautifully and elongates a short or thick neck. But depending on its cut, different body shapes have different width of scoop.

A wide or large scooped neckline on a shirt, for example, tends to flatter women with narrow shoulders since it makes the shoulders appear wider. It also fits better for smaller chests or women with athletic body builds. As for bustier ladies or those with broad shoulders, they can do a smaller scoop to disguise their large area.

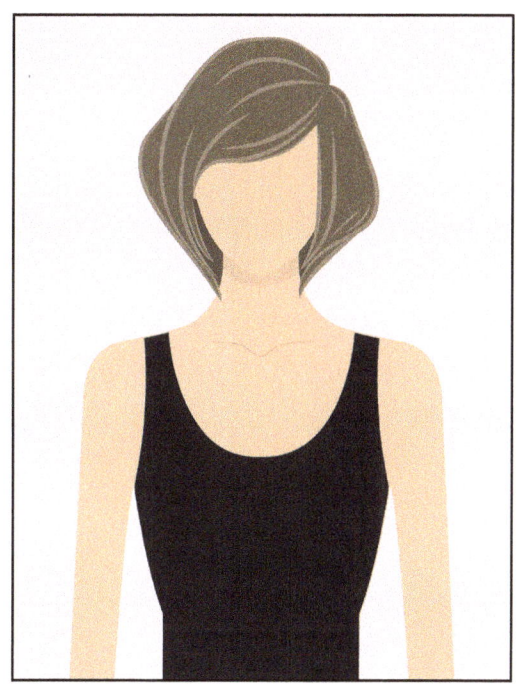

The scoop neckline is best recommended for:

- short neck, oblong face shape, or narrow shoulders, as it gives the illusion of a longer and wider look.
- the pear body shape, as it creates a balanced look between smaller upper and larger lower body part.
- to create the illusion of a larger bust.
- hourglass body shapes, as it will give the illusion of a bit larger shoulder line, since theirs are equal with their hips.

Necklace Suggestions

To bring emphasis down, the scoop neckline is best paired with a feature necklace that mimics the scoop. Fill in the space with multiple strands of beads or larger scale pendants. A long plunging chain necklace can also be effective for drawing the eyes to the centre of the body.

Sweetheart Neckline

A sweetheart neckline forms two curves like a type of heart shape at the bust-line that rise over the underarms and reach high over the breasts.

This neckline has a shape to provide considerable coverage to the breasts. This works well in accentuating cleavage.

The best thing about this shape is it visually elongates the face and provides proportional balance to the overall silhouette. Women with a round back and shoulders must avoid the sweetheart neckline as it will draw attention to the roundness.

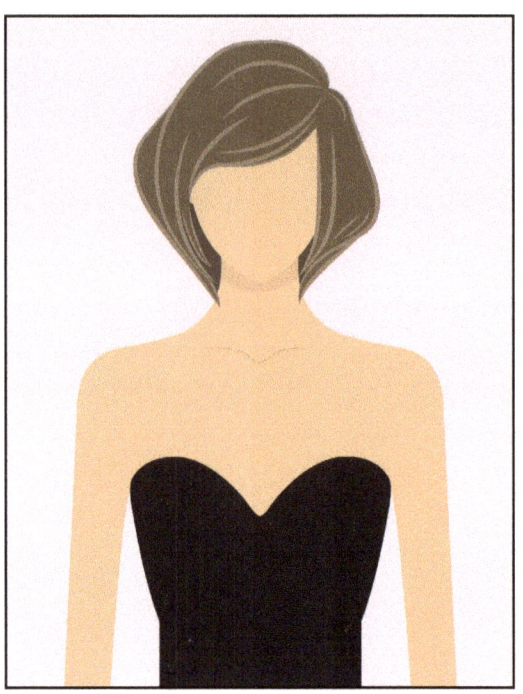

The sweetheart neckline suits almost every body shape and size but is best recommended for:

- busty ladies who want to accentuate cleavage, but larger body shapes will look better when having straps or shoulders with this neckline.
- those with a short chin and neck.
- angular face shape, as it balances the contours of the sweetheart.
- petite women with small breasts and narrow shoulders, who can wear them to give the illusion of more curves.

Necklace Suggestions

Since this neckline has a flirty style, opt for a statement necklace to give a modern touch, or chunky necklaces and pendant necklaces, which can be simple or bold. A curved necklace that has width will balance the open décolletage of this neckline.

Straight-Across (Strapless) Neckline

The straight-across neckline is of the most favourite among women and is widely used for cocktail parties or special occasions. Because it shows great value around the neck and arms area, a strapless top tends to be most flattering on women who have wider shoulders and a small bust line. This neckline doesn't fit all body types because it leaves the shoulders and arms fully displayed.

Women with small to medium breasts, and preferably slim or well-built, take the most benefit from this look. Wear a strapless bra with great support. Stay clear from wearing clear bra straps.

The petite figure can also invest in this neckline to give a longer and taller silhouette. Strapless styles also help to elongate the neck.

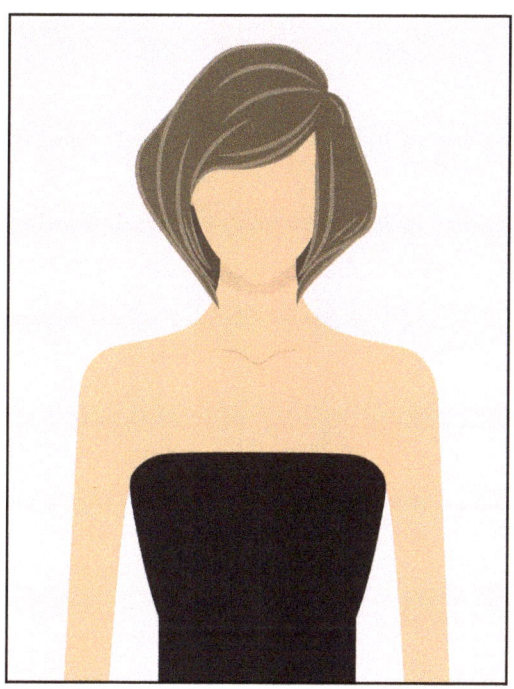

The straight-across (strapless) neckline is best recommended for:

- well-toned arms.
- good shoulders.
- medium bust.
- long neck.

Necklace Suggestions

This neckline looks great with short pendants, leaving your lovely décolletage bare. For a more dramatic effect, opt for statement necklaces or chunky ones. If you want to go for a long necklace, choose a simple necklace with small beads, so that it won't compete with the strapless look.

Halter Neckline

The halter neckline attracts attention to the centre of the body. Halters are perfect for women with tall and/or broad shoulders. They cut broad shoulder lines and also add curves.

The shape of the halter-neck is incredibly flattering, and also very flexible that it can be worn well by almost all body shapes, particularly for those with an hourglass body shape.

For the busty ladies, especially if they also have bulky arms, pay more attention since this neckline also creates the impression of greater volume and will make you look wider than you actually are.

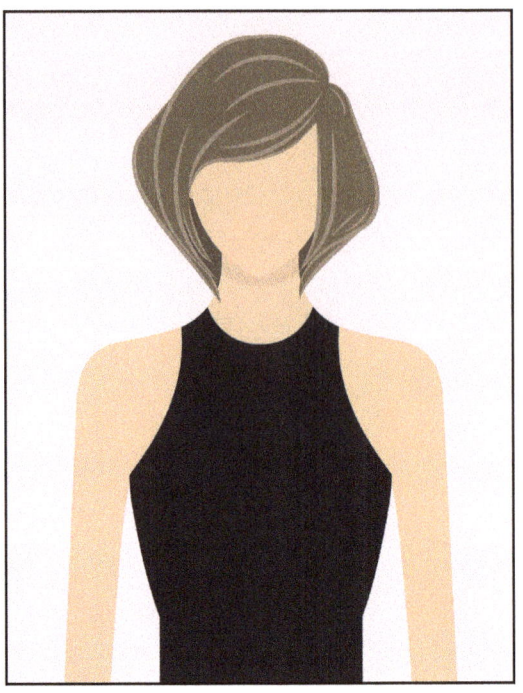

The halter neckline suits almost every body type and size, but is best recommended for:

- good or well-toned arms.
- good shoulders.
- average- to small-busted ladies.

Necklace Suggestions

Pairing a necklace with a halter neckline can be tough. These shapes create a narrow V-neck, so look for a narrow pendant with a sharper end. If you're wearing a halter neckline with a keyhole at the bust or spacing in the fabric, you're better off not wearing a necklace at all because it creates enough attention already. Stick with beautiful earrings or an upper arm band.

Boat Neckline

The boat neck is also known as princess or bateau neckline. It is great for offsetting wide hips since it softly follows the curve of the collarbone and tends to make shoulders visually wider. Generally, this neckline looks best on women with long necks and smaller heads because the style can make both look wider. Be mindful if you have broad shoulders because it can make your shoulders look even broader.

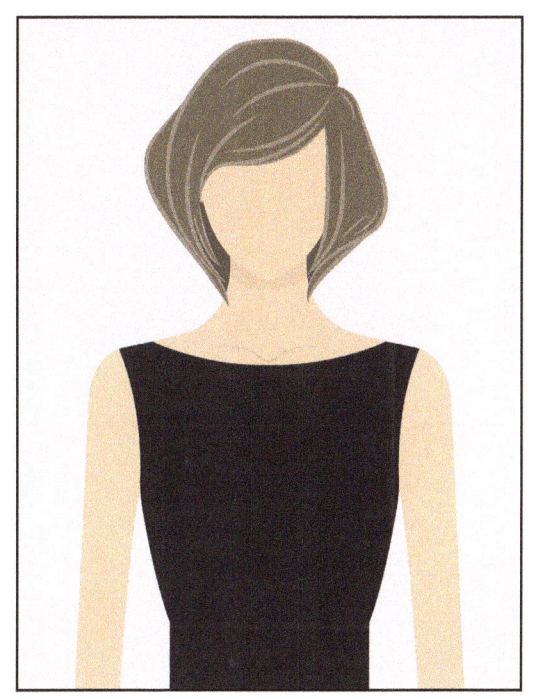

It enhances the chest area and is great for ladies with a small chest. But if you have a short, thick neck or double chin, be careful with this high-necked style, as it will only draw attention to these areas.

The boat neckline is best recommended for:

- ➤ the hourglass body shape, as it covers the arms elegantly and comfortably.
- ➤ ladies with average to small bust, as it gives the illusion of larger breasts.
- ➤ narrow shoulders, particularly if reinforced with small shoulder pads.
- ➤ the rectangle body shape, as it balances the shoulders.
- ➤ oblong face, as it cuts the length of the facial structure.
- ➤ long neck and beautiful collarbone.
- ➤ women with bulky arms, who can wear a boat neckline with a shoulder cap or strap, which gives a bit more cover and gives the illusion of smaller arms; even an added cap sleeve will work very well when in a darker fabric colour.

Necklace Suggestions

This neckline draws a lot of attention and do not need a necklace. If you feel you must wear something, it's best to pair it with a longer pendant necklace. A long string or two of beads is ideal for this neckline. For the much lower boat neckline, you can choose a collar necklace.

Round Neckline

The round neckline basically suits all body types, but women with a large bust, a short neck, or a double chin should pay attention to its scoop, as it can emphasize those areas and make them look wider. Because it extends high up on the chest, it decreases the amount of exposed skin between the chin and chest, making the neckline look shorter and thicker.

This neckline is classic, simple, and super versatile. They are available in a wide range of styles, and there are many different ways to wear them. The round face or double chin must rather avoid this neckline style entirely because it will draw attention to the roundness of the face.

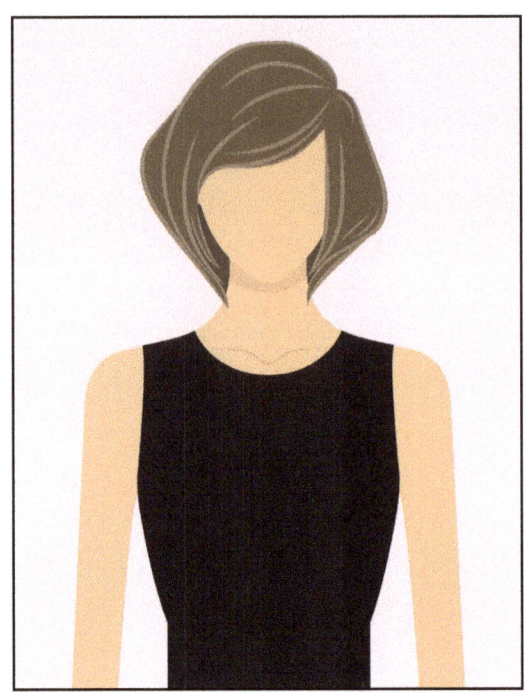

The round neckline suits almost every body shape and size, but is best recommended for:

- ladies with average to small bust, as it gives the illusion of larger breasts.
- oblong face and rectangular face shapes, as it cuts the length of the face.
- a long neck.

Necklace Suggestions

You can easily wear a bib necklace, a pendant necklace, a collar necklace, or just about any style necklace that you'd like. For the shorter neck, a short necklace can compete with the neckline; therefore, a long necklace will look better. Charms or tassels dangling at the ends will look beautiful.

Cowl Neckline

A cowl neck is a draped neckline in rounded folds that hangs in a loosely fashionable way. It can be either high-necked or open to reveal more skin around the neck.

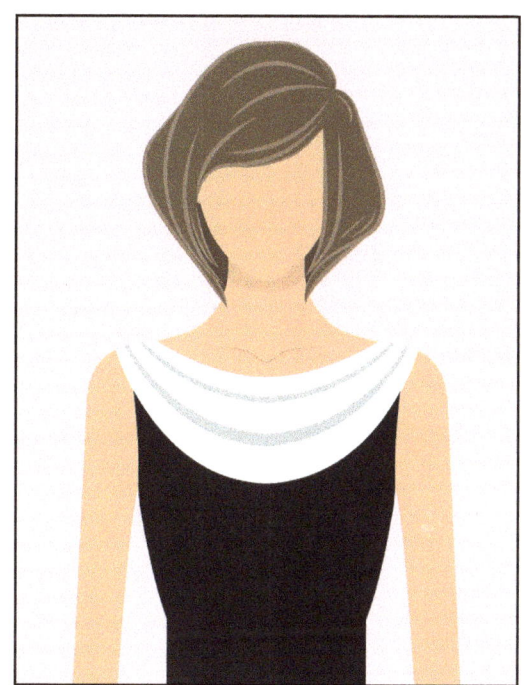

This draped neckline can generally flatter a variety of body shapes. It creates a leaner appearance, and can also add volume to a smaller chest. It is best avoided by ladies with a larger bust, or a fuller figure, due to the extra inches added by the excess fabric.

Petite ladies should choose a smaller cowl neckline, to avoid being swamped by too many layers.

The cowl neckline suits almost every body shape and size, but is best recommended for:

- ladies with small to medium bust.
- lean body shapes because it creates extra volume.
- long neck figures since it adds volume, making the neck look shorter.
- those whose head is bigger in proportion to the upper body, as the cowl will give proportional balance.

Necklace Suggestions

Wearing a necklace with a cowl-neck can be tricky since the neckline has such a bold, distinctive look already. Wear something thin and small, which is one colour. If you really do not have confidence to pair it right, you'd be better off not wearing a necklace at all; wear beautiful earrings instead.

Off-Shoulder Neckline

The off-shoulder neckline sits off the shoulders or below them and runs along the collarbone. They are similar to boat necklines in that they generally cut across the figure nearly horizontally, but significantly lower, below the shoulders and collarbone.

Off-shoulders come in several different styles. Some expose both shoulders at once, while some expose only one shoulder. But generally, these are best for the well-endowed, as it enhances a flattering yet elegant effect around the bust area.

Women with a small bust will look good if the off-shoulder have a frill or band hanging down to give the illusion of a larger bust area.

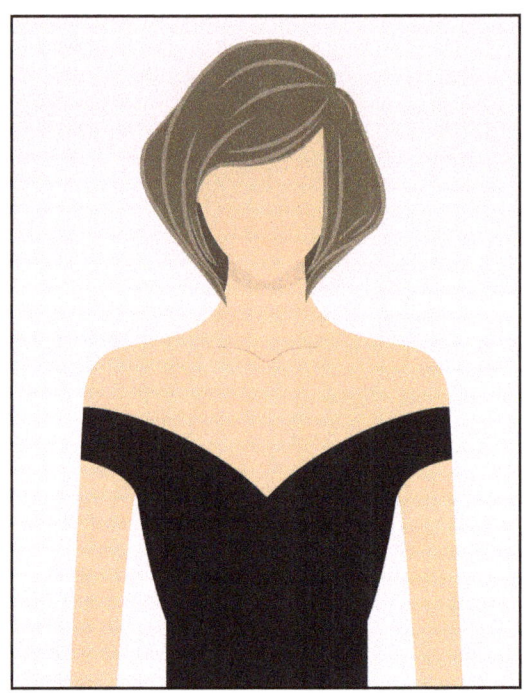

Off-shoulder necklines suit almost every body shape and size, but is best recommended for:

- the pear body shape or those with narrow shoulders, as the off-shoulder neckline gives shoulders a broader look.
- pear body shapes to balance the top and bottom part; the skirt must be straight or an A-frame to create a slimming effect on the hips and bottom.
- showing off beautiful clavicles and bosom.

Necklace Suggestions

Similar to the boat neck, this neckline is best paired with a longer necklace. However, because this neckline sits below the collarbone, wearing it with a choker or collar necklace is also a beautiful option.

Asymmetrical Neckline (One Shoulder)

The asymmetrical neckline gives a dramatic look, and depending on the material used, a one-shoulder neckline can be elegant and formal, informal and casual, or sleek and modern.

Generally, the one-shoulder neckline acts like the strapless and off-shoulder neckline, which add more volume around the bust area. Wear a strapless bra with great support, coverage, and comfort.

Women with a large bust area should pay more attention when wearing an asymmetrical garment as well as women with broad shoulders since the asymmetrical line creates the impression of greater volume.

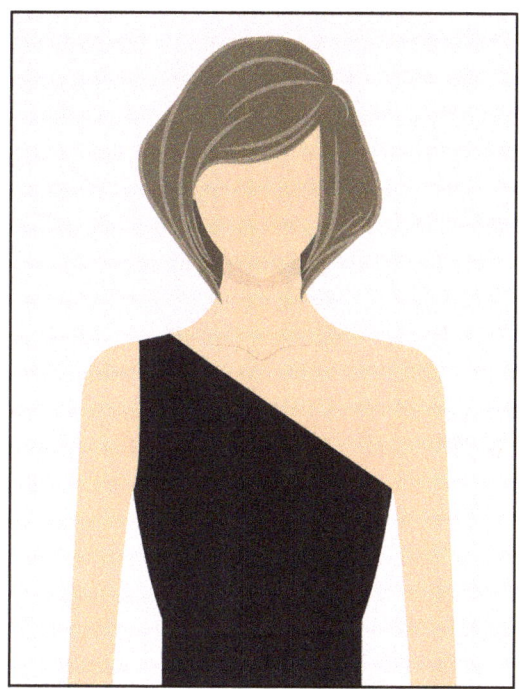

The asymmetric neckline suits almost every body shape and size, but is best recommended for:

- women with narrow shoulders and thin arms, who will look great with this neckline, since it can give a wider effect around the shoulders and upper-arm area.
- those with a long neck and nice collarbone, who will also benefit from wearing this neckline since it accentuates the collarbone, and disguises a, long thin neck.
- those with small to medium bust area.

Necklace Suggestions

This is another tricky neckline to pair a necklace with. A long string with beads of different sizes and shapes can work well, but the key is to make sure the necklace is long enough to clear at least 2 inches above or below the neckline. If the necklace competes with the asymmetrical line, avoid wearing it.

Backless Neckline

The backless neckline is flattering and alluring. It works well for the thin to medium-sized body shapes and those with a great back.

For the plus size, try to choose a garment that is less open and has a higher cut. Avoid leaving the unwanted parts exposed, especially around the waist.

On the other hand, all suggestions aside, if you are confident with the outfit you want to pull off, it will work. Always look for comfort in the most elegant way.

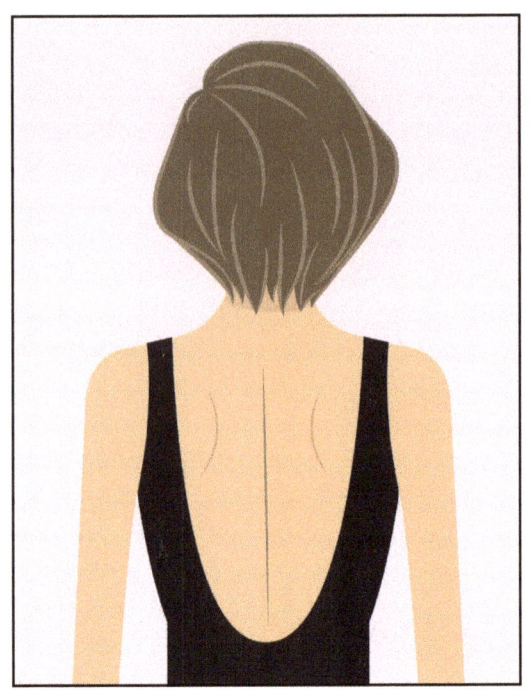

The backless neckline is best recommended for:

- those with tall and lean body shapes, who must take care not to show the whole back or go down too low because it can attract attention to their height.
- good arms for the sleeveless, backless garment.
- good, clean back and shoulders.
- small to medium bust area.

Necklace Suggestions

When the neckline in front is higher and up to the bottom of the neck, the necklace is best to end at least 2 inches below the front neckline or the lowest point between the boobs. For a lower front neckline, a short necklace will look better because it will not compete with the backless line.

Illusion Neckline

The illusion neckline can be thought of as featuring two necklines in one: a strapless sweetheart neckline and a sheer panel of fabric (typically lace, tulle, organza, or other), which attaches to the bodice, usually at the waistline, and extends upward, forming the second, higher neckline.

It is a classic and elegant style, showing just enough skin, making this a beautiful fusion of modern style and conservative style. It is the popular strapless neckline with the added support of cut-in sleeves. Some may find the netted fabrics of the illusion neckline scratchy or uncomfortable. It's easily solved; make sure your gown features a soft, netted fabric or lace.

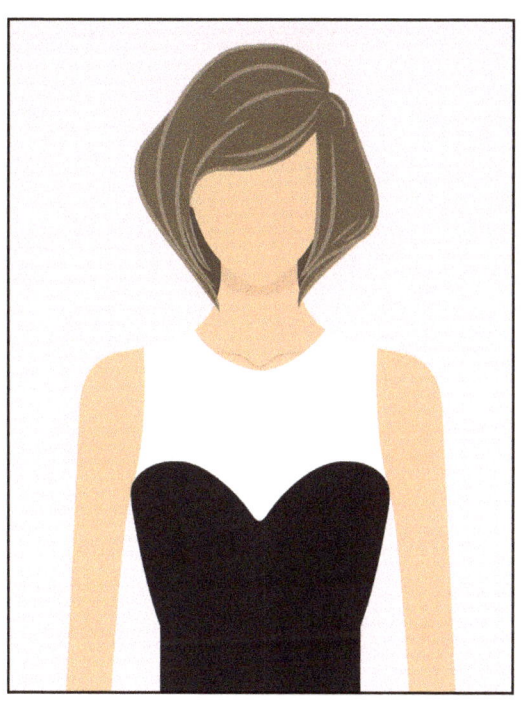

The illusion neckline suits almost every body shape and size, but is best recommended for:

- well-toned or good arms and good shoulders when the illusion shoulder lines are cut-in sleeves.
- ladies with small to medium bust, as the round lines around the boobs gives the illusion that the boobs are bigger.
- oblong face shapes, as the higher round neckline of the lace cuts the length of the facial structure.
- long necks, where the higher round illusion will make it appear shorter.

Necklace Suggestions

Usually, the lace makes an interesting pattern which draws enough attention, and there is no need to double up with a necklace. You can always wear interesting earrings and hairclips.

Spaghetti Straps Neckline

Spaghetti straps can be attached to a few different necklines, including the sweatheart neckline, V-neckline, off-shoulder neckline, halter neckline, straight-across neckline, cowl neckline, backless neckline, and a scoop neckline.

The main purpose is to give extra support, but is also used to create interesting variation to the standard necklines.

While the body shapes with bigger shoulders and arms would be careful in wearing straight-across (strapless) and sweatheart necklines, which expose areas and make it appear larger, it would be safer to add spaghetti straps, that will add vertical lines and give more of a slimming effect.

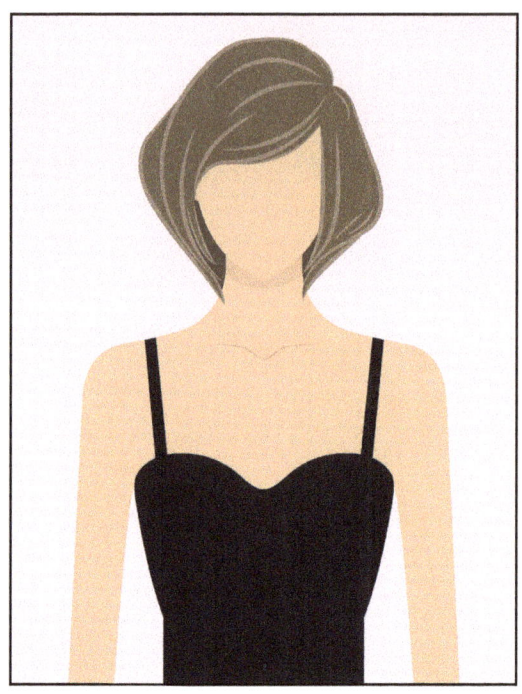

Spaghetti straps suit almost every body shape and size, but is best recommended for:

- good shoulders and arms.
- ladies with small to medium bust.
- for wearing with the correct neckline that fits your face shape.
- changing the look of the original neckline, therefore, look at the new neckline it creates, and use the suggestions in this book to determine if it will still fit you well; for example, when you add straps to the halter neckline, it changes to a round neckline close to the face.

Necklace Suggestions

Depending on the gap, the best size for the necklace is short to medium, halfway between the clavicles and the neckline. The halter and cowl necklines create enough interest, and you do not need to double up with a necklace. Wear beautiful earrings instead.

Queen Anne Neckline

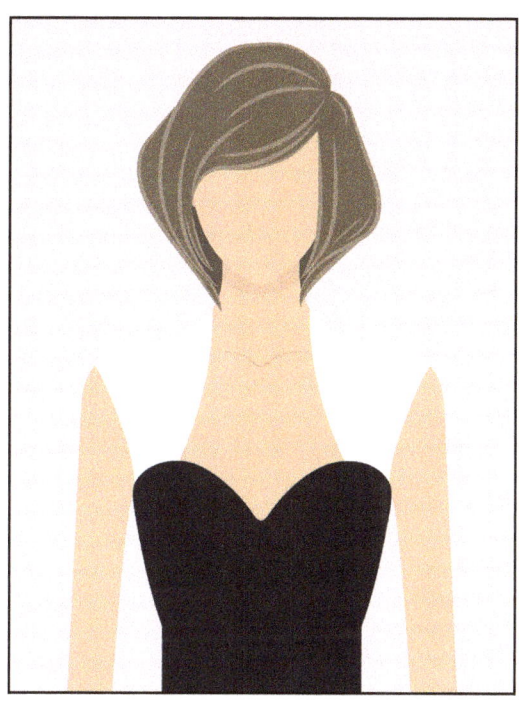

The Queen Anne neckline opens up the area and elongates the neck, which is ideal for petite ladies and anyone with a shorter neck. The high neck at the back of the dress and the thicker straps across the shoulders make this a modest choice as well as a glamorous one.

There are different patterns of the Queen Anne and can also be raised at the back of the neck and head.

The Queen Anne neckline gives the wearer an elegant, formal, and sophisticated look. It is a very popular neckline to use in a wedding dress. Women with a round back and shoulders, for whom the sweetheart neckline is not suited, can wear the Queen Anne neckline as an alternative.

The Queen Anne neckline suits almost every body shape and size, but is best recommended for:

- ➢ short chin and neck, because it opens up the décolletage area.
- ➢ angular face shape, as it balances the contours of the sweetheart.
- ➢ petite women with small breasts and narrow shoulders, who may wear them to show more curves if the dress or top has bra infills.

Necklace Suggestions

The Queen Anne has a very elegant look. It is better not to wear a necklace, but if you feel you have to, it should be very small; for example, a small pearl pendant. You can also wear beautiful earrings and hairclips to make up for not wearing any necklace.

Shoulder Lines and Creating Optical Illusion with Style

Creating Balance with Shoulder Lines

In order for our figure to appear balanced, the shoulders need to be the widest part of our body. Ideally, the shoulders should be 2-3 centimetres wider than the hips to allow the lines of clothes to fall loosely over the hips from the shoulders.

The quickest, cheapest, and most effective method to achieve visual figure balance is the appropriate use of shoulder pads. They should not look big or bulky, or too small that they hardly make any difference. Another important part is selecting the correct fit of the shoulders and sleeves. This will create the balance that your body shape needs. For example, narrow shoulders need to appear wider, and broad shoulders need to appear narrower. With the lean and rectangle body shapes, which are basically straight, you want the shoulders to appear slightly wider than the hips.

Ask the following questions to determine if the balance in the figure is working:

- Does the shoulder line balance the waist, hips, and thighs?
- Do you need to use shoulder pads or line design, or both, to improve your shoulder line?
- Does your body shape need shoulder pads to straighten a dropped -shoulder line to improve posture?

Sleeves

The sleeves of a garment must not be too tight, big, or bulky, which will add unwanted weight to your overall look, unless your body shape is lean and you want to give the illusion of extra weight. The shoulder of a garment affects the look of your entire silhouette. The seam of the shoulder can give your shoulders the definition of shape they may lack. A woman with a very large bust can use the shoulder seam to draw the attention away from her bust. For example, by wearing the set-in sleeve, you'll draw the eyes up and down, whereas with a puff- or dropped shoulder sleeve, it will give the illusion of being wider. For broad and square shoulders, keep the edge of the garment on the shoulder bone as a set-in sleeve, or wear a raglan sleeve, which draws the eye away from the broadness.

Following are a few popular sleeve lines and which body shapes will benefit from wearing them.

The Most Common Sleeve Styles

Set-In Sleeve

This is the most popular sleeve style. It is flattering for all body types where the fit is balanced to make the shoulders slightly broader than the hips. In the case of the pear body shape, the seam of the shoulders can be extended to make the shoulders look a bit broader.

Body shapes that will benefit from the set-in sleeve: all body shapes except the pear/triangle body shape, which needs the shoulder line a bit wider.

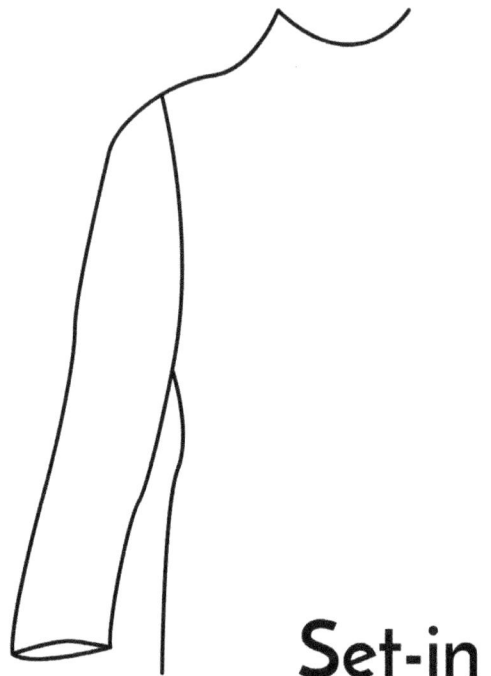

Raglan Sleeve

The raglan creates the appearance of a longer arm. Elongating the arm helps to create a slimming effect, while also breaking up the shoulder line. This is a sleeve to shrink broad shoulders. The diagonal lines minimize a large bust area and can disguise a flat chest.

Body shapes that will benefit from the raglan sleeve: all body shapes.

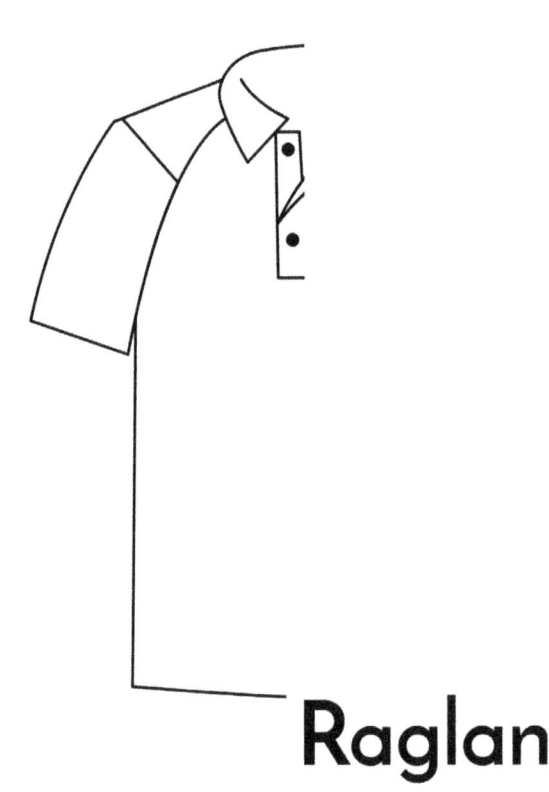

Batwing Sleeve

Batwing sleeves have a deep armhole that extends and tapers towards the wrist, creating a silhouette that does, indeed, look like a batwing. They are comfortable to wear and surprisingly will work for many body shapes. The only drawback of wearing this sleeve is that you cannot wear anything over it.

Body shapes that will benefit from the batwing sleeve: all body shapes.

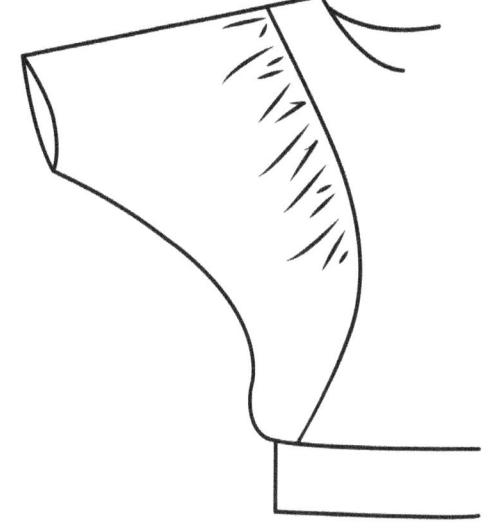

Batwing

Petal Sleeve

The petal sleeve is two pieces of fabric crossing over each other, creating a look that's soft and feminine. Depending on the fabric used, thicker and more firm fabrics will make the shoulder line appear wider, whereas a soft, flowy type will form around the arm and add a bit lesser width.

Body shapes that will benefit from the petal sleeve: all body shapes, but take in consideration the type of fabric and length of the sleeve for the inverted-triangle body shape, as it can create more width.

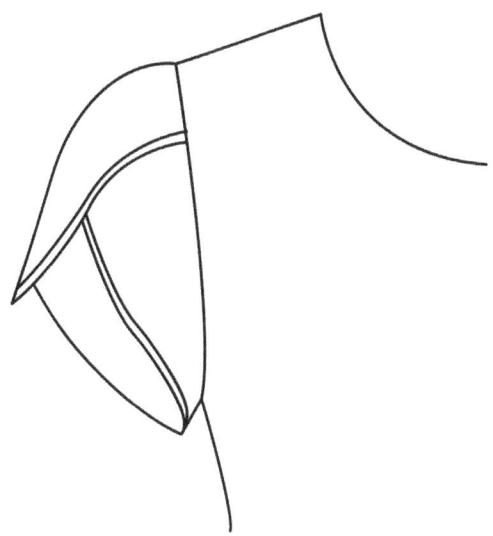

Petal

Puff Sleeve

The puff sleeve of a woman's garment is gathered at the shoulders and can be caught in at the cuff to create an inflated, puffy effect. It is combined with different sleeve lengths from short to full lengths. The extra volume makes shoulders quite literally larger. Women with small arms and shoulders will benefit.

Body shapes that will benefit from the set-in sleeve: triangle/pear, lean, hourglass, petite, and rectangle.

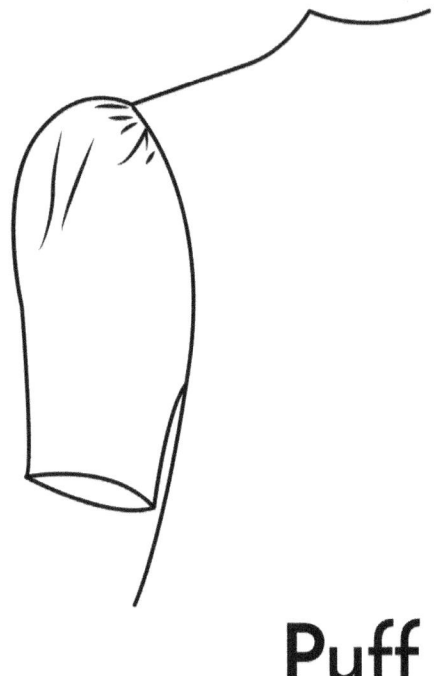

Puff

Cap Sleeve

The cap sleeve sits directly on the shoulder and can have a slimming effect on the forearm. It extends the shoulders, therefore balancing it with the waist, hips, and thighs.

Body shapes that will benefit from the cap sleeve: all body shapes.

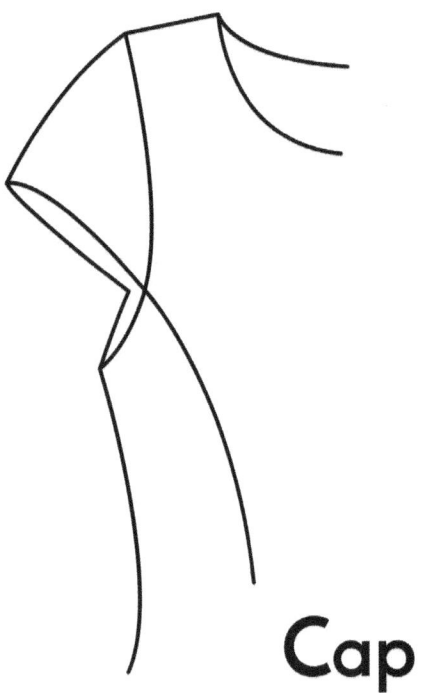

Cap

Dropped-Shoulder Sleeve

The dropped-shoulder pattern gives a broader look to the shoulder line. The straight line encourages the eyes to carry on looking.

Body shapes that will benefit from the dropped-shoulder sleeve: triangle/pear, lean, hourglass, round/apple, rectangle, and the slim petite who wears high heels.

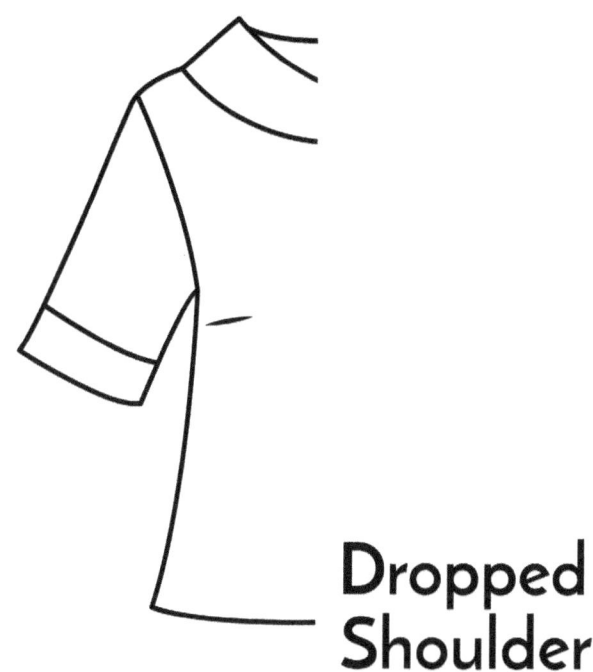

Dropped Shoulder

Cut-In Sleeveless

It is the most difficult sleeve style for most body shapes to wear well because it requires good or toned arms and shoulders. This sleeve is very effective on the perfectly balanced shoulders. The inverted triangle body shape will benefit most from this sleeve, as it takes the eye away from the broad shoulders and gives the illusion of smaller.

Body shapes that will benefit from the cut-in sleeve: inverted triangle, rectangle, lean, petite, hourglass.

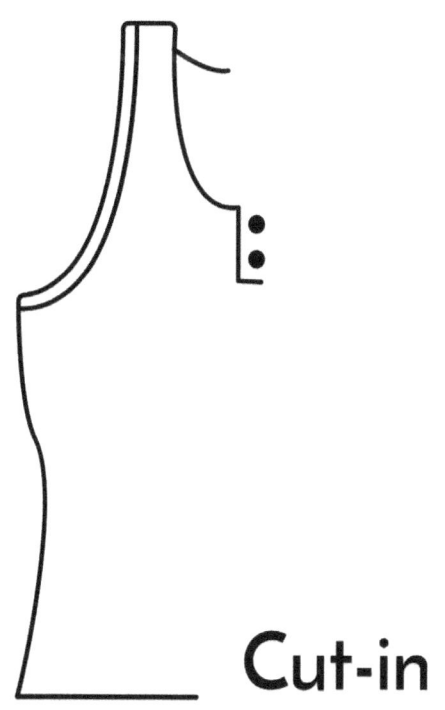

Cut-in

How to Create Optical Illusion with Style

Legs

Ladies with very long legs can wear trousers with turn-ups. The horizontal lines that the turn-ups create will break the length of the legs a bit. Jackets should end slightly below the crotch when viewed from the front. Avoid jackets ending in the waist as it will expose long legs.

Short legs must avoid turn-ups on their trousers because it will make the legs appear shorter. Wear high heels to give the illusion of height; at least a 5 centimetre heels will make a difference. Keep your suit jackets relatively short, no lower than the crotch and preferably at the break of the leg. Blouses and over tops should be shorter than your suit jacket for a balanced look.

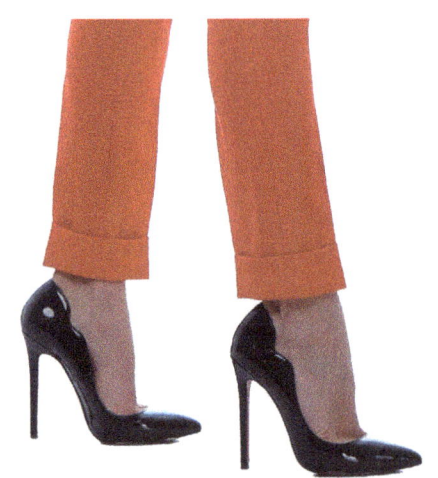

Average length legs can wear turn-ups or no turn-ups, and the best suit jacket length with trousers is at the crotch.

Heavy Thighs, Hips, and Bottom

The easiest way to disguise large thighs is to wear A-line skirts and dresses with a slight fullness to provide easy camouflage. Avoid trousers that taper at the ankle because it will emphasize the heavy thighs. Tight-fitting trousers will also reveal any heaviness. The best trousers to wear when you have large thighs are straight pipes.

The pear/triangle body shape, who has wide hips, must avoid full gathered skirts, hip pockets, and horizontal lines on skirts and trousers, which will add more volume. Keep the skirts straight to an A-line pattern (the skirt becomes wider to the hemline in straight fabric pattern without any pleats from the waistband), in darker-coloured fabrics. Trousers must have straight line patterns on the hips without any pockets or pleats.

Women with narrow hips can wear everything that adds more width to the hips. The hourglass body shape, which has a tiny waistline and large hips and breasts, must be careful not to pull the waist in too tight, as it can draw attention to the larger hips and breasts.

Bottoms that are too heavy, flat, or slim can be easily fixed by wearing an A-line skirt, pleated skirt, or dress to camouflage. Be conscious of a tight-fitted jacket around the bottom if you do not want to accentuate your curves. Wear short jackets with straight lines ending just above the crest of the bottom. Never wear a jacket that is too long for you because it will only make your legs look short and your body heavy.

Waistlines

Figures with a small to medium waistline can wear large belts or waistbands. To make your waist appear smaller, you can cheat by raising the waistline a bit above your real waistline. The round and plus-size body shapes will not be able to use this trick, but there are other clever ways discussed in this book.

There is no point to attract attention to a large waistline. If you must wear a belt, keep it narrow and the same colour as the garment it is worn over. When it matches the colour of the skirt or trousers, it will draw the eyes up to your beautiful face. This way you will not draw too much attention to your wide waist.

Short-waisted women should wear narrow belts the same colour as the outfit to draw attention away from the short upper body. On the other hand, wearing no belts may be better. Optical illusion tricks can make the upper body appear longer; for example, vertical lines, diagonal lines, and lighter-coloured bodices of the garments. Darker skirts and trousers give the illusion of the bottom part being smaller and shorter (hips and legs), to bring balance. Shirts and jackets must not stop at the waist but rather end at the crotch to balance the top half with the bottom half of the body.

Long-waisted women can wear medium- to large-sized belts in the middle so that most of the belt is positioned above the true waistline. Wear horizontal lines and darker colours on the upper body to minimize the long upper body (measured from the waist to the top of the head). Lighter colours, and vertical or diagonal lines in the skirts and trousers will bring a balancing effect between the upper and lower body. Jackets can stop in the waistline to break the upper body's length a bit.

The Different Widths of Belts

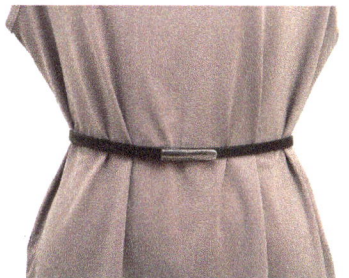
Small belt.

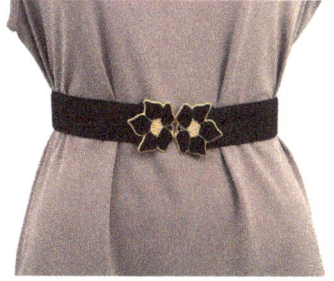
Medium belt.

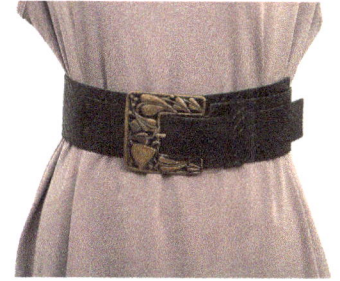
Large belt.

Arms

To determine if your arm is long, average or short, let your arm hang at your side while you are looking in the mirror. Your elbow should be at the waist. If your knuckle aligns with your crotch, you have an average arm.

Long Arms

If you have long arms, a wide cuff at the wrist shortens the look of your arm. A woman with long arms often has trouble finding sleeves that are long enough. Don't overlook the possibility of adding lace cuffs to the garment sleeves, even in a contrasting colour.

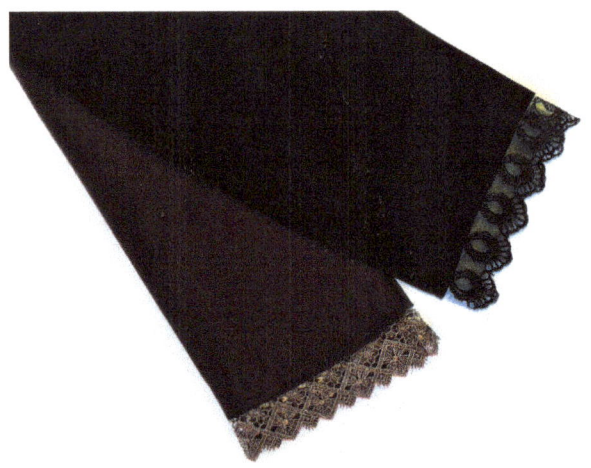

Example of added lace cuffs to jackets for too-long arms.

Short Arms

Women with short arms should avoid a cuff. The three-quarter-length sleeves work best on a short woman or one with short arms.

Short sleeves

The short sleeve usually looks better if it falls 2-3 centimetres (1 inch) above or below the furthest point of the bust-line, rather than right at the point of the bust. If you have a small bust, it may not matter.

A short sleeve ending just above the elbow can look matronly, especially if it has a rolled cuff or if your arms are heavy. In high-style clothing, this sleeve length can be attractive if you are slim and tall with average to long arms. Women with heavy arms must avoid long sleeves that are tight or clingy; this will accentuate the bulkiness.

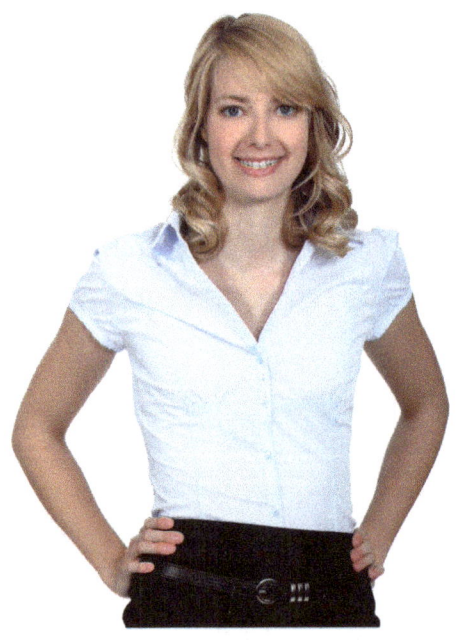

Bust

The bra that you are wearing determines how an outfit displays on you. Take a good look at yourself to be sure your bra is doing its job. Many women make the mistake of buying bra cups too small or too big, and the band to large. Shop for a bra that fits comfortably around your rib-cage with cups that hold the entire breast tissue firmly but also not too tight. Bra straps should not fall off the shoulders if you are wearing a bra that's the right size. The larger the size of the bra cup, the wider the straps should be to give adequate support to the breasts and back.

Tips for women who are conscious of their large bust:

- Avoid horizontal lines in stripes, patterns, seams, and piping at bust level. Rather wear plain fabrics over the bust, and style up the lower part of the figure with vertical lines, pockets, pleats, lighter- and brighter-coloured fabrics, etc.
- Avoid sleeve lengths ending at the point of the bust level, but rather 2-3 centimetres above or under.
- Do not wear garments that have pleats or smocking patterns in the bodice of the garment; it will add more fullness around the bust.
- A tight-fitted bodice will also accentuate the bust.
- Wear V-necklines with lapels and open collars, which have a slimming effect on the bust-line.
- Avoid high-waisted skirts, trousers, and dresses and low-scoop necklines that will reveal more.

Bra Tips and Facts

Your bra is the most important garment, and it is easy to forget or neglect to update it. It is hard to remember how a great bra should look and feel like, if you have worn the same one for a long time.

For the most comfortable and perfect fit, you should put your bra on as follows: Put each arm through the straps one-by-one and place over each shoulder. Then lift the cups over the breasts. Use opposite hands to pull each breast into the cup. Secure the bra clasp on your back, and use opposite hands again to make sure the nipples are in the centre of each cup.

The band around your back must be firm but not tight, as it provides 85 per cent of the support to your entire breast tissue. The straps should be firm and not digging into your shoulders, leaving red press marks. They provide around 15 per cent of the overall support of lifting your breast tissue.

The underwire must encase your bust perfectly and sit just underneath your breast tissue, at the sides towards the armpit. When you raise your arms above your head, the underwire should not move forward or upward and should sit flat on your rib-cage.

The centre of the bra must sit comfortably against your sternum, separating breast tissue with the exact width your breasts sit apart from one another. Your breasts must not spill out over the top of the bra cup and should fill the inside of the bra cup. When you slip the bra straps off the shoulders, your breasts should still sit in the correct place because of the correct band and cup size.

In the correctly fitting bra, your nipples should be placed exactly halfway between your shoulder line and elbow. A quality bra should last anywhere between thirty-six to forty-eight months. Ideally, your bra should be so comfortable that you do not even realize that you are wearing one.

Caring Tips for Bras to Last Longer

Hand-wash your bras in lukewarm water with liquid laundry soap that is a softer soap, such as liquid laundry detergent.

Hang bras to dry away from direct sunlight. For example, hang it on a portable clothing rack with the centre of the bra (between the two cups) resting directly over the line or bar, in the shade, which can be the side of your house or an undercover area.

When your bras are dry, hang it in your wardrobe over clothes hangers so that the centre of the bra is resting directly over the hangers. This way the straps will not get overstretched on hangers or squashed in a drawer. It will also air them out in between wearing.

A good portion of bras are made out of elastic, and it is best to have at least four to five quality bras so that you can alternate from day to day to give the fabrication a chance to rest and restore its elasticity.

Our body heat warms up the bra, which causes the elastic to gradually stretch. To give the elastic time to recover, do not wear a bra on consecutive days. Body salts also cause wear and tear to the bra fabric. This is the natural ageing process that we do not have control over.

Heat destroys the small elastic fibres in bras; therefore, do not dry your bras in the tumble drier. If you live in a cold and humid environment, let the bras first drip dry over the clothes rack and only put damp bras through the tumble drier on low heat and not for longer than five minutes. If it's still a bit damp after this process, hang it in your wardrobe with some space between each side, to dry it completely overnight.

NO PAIN OR SLIPPAGE
NO SPILLAGE
NO POKING
SNUG, BUT NO PAIN

Band is Parallel to Waist
Band Rides Up
GOOD FIT
BAD FIT

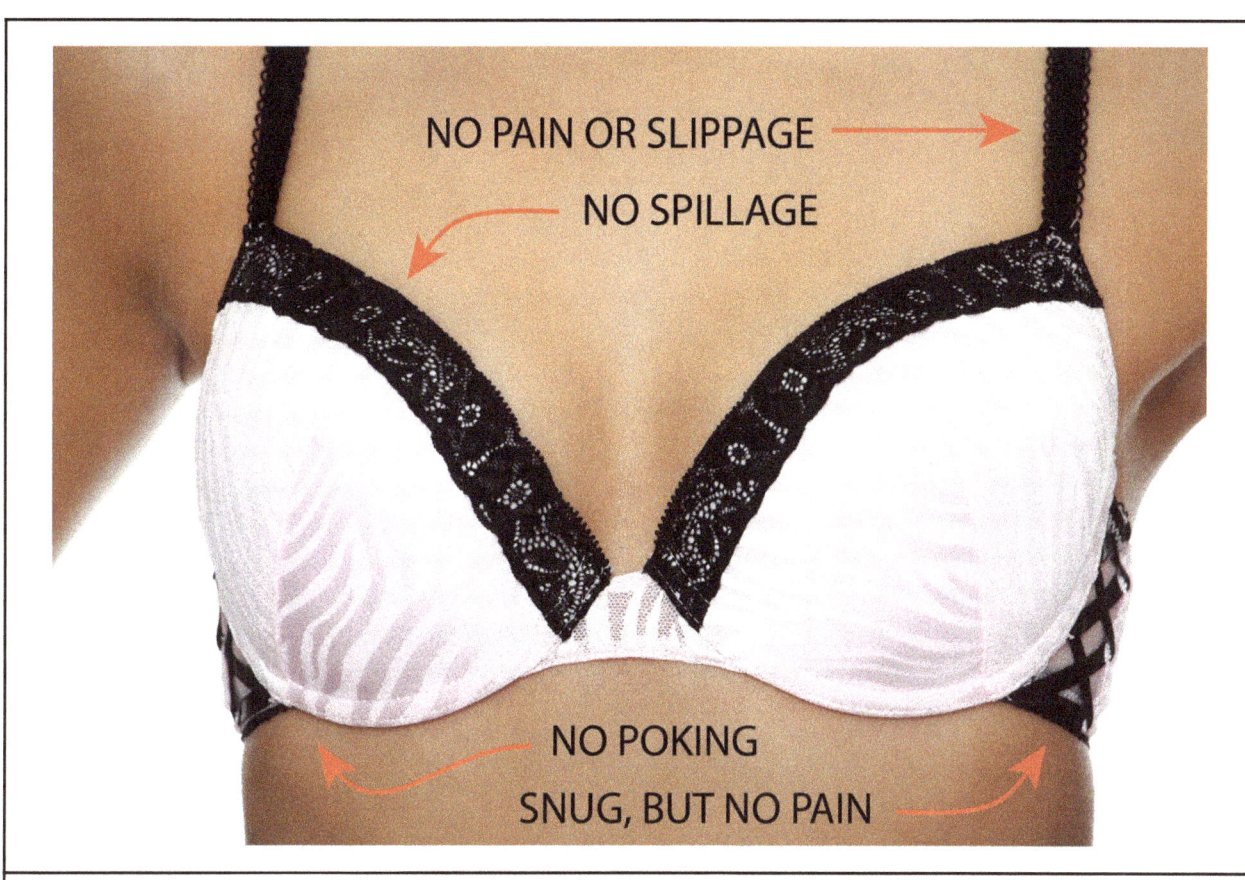

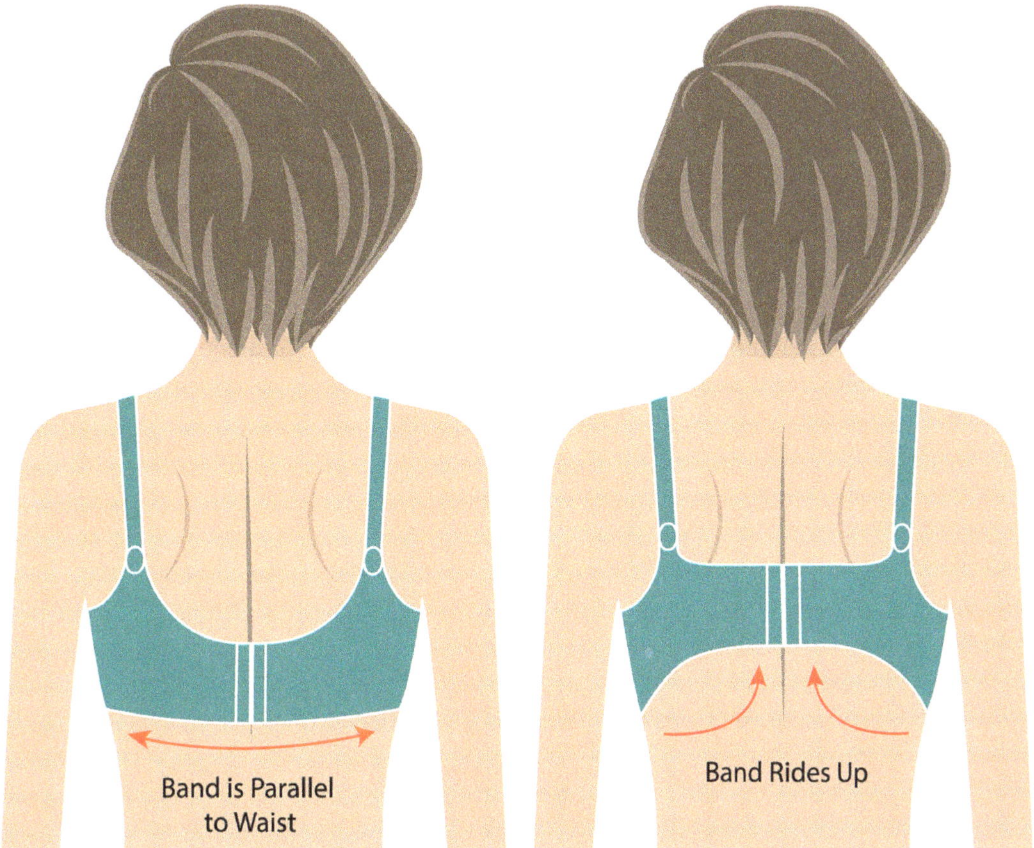

Height

Short women look especially good in high-waisted clothes and shorter-length jackets. A three-quarter sleeve and accessories or trim near the face will draw the eye up.

Women who are tall and slim can wear most styles. Tall women can wear heavier fabrics, more fullness or pleats, and low-waisted styles. If you are taller than 1.74 centimetres (5.7 feet), avoid high-waisted lines, including short waist-length jackets. These lines increase the illusion of height and sometimes make a very tall woman look tiny on the upper body.

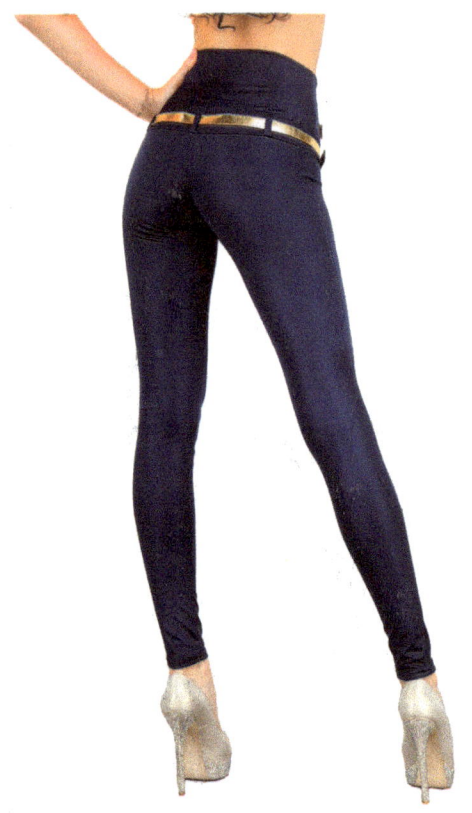
High-waisted pants.

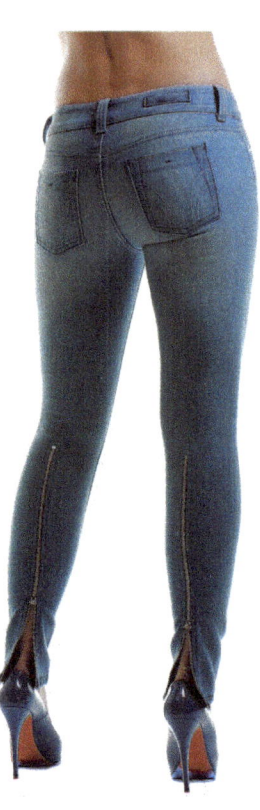
Low-waisted pants.

Weight

If you are too slim or overweight, you have a special need to create an illusion with clothing styles, lines, colours, and fabric print. In either case, you should avoid clothes that are too tight and revealing. Too-tight clothes will accentuate both underweight and overweight figures.

The Most Slimming Techniques in Style

- Use vertical lines and diagonal lines in fabric print, seams, and pattern.
- Avoid horizontal lines and details.
- Darker colours are more slimming than lighter colours.

- Plain cuts are more slimming than patterns with pleats and pockets.
- Wearing your true dress size is more slimming than wearing one or two dress sizes bigger.
- Small to medium accessories, like handbags and cosmetic jewellery, are more slimming than large to extra-large accessories.
- Wearing underwear that fits you well gives your figure a beautiful shape, and you'll look slimmer than, for example, wearing a worn-out or no bra. Too small underwear, again, creates bulges that can be seen through the clothes.
- Wear the correct length for hemlines or jackets, sleeves, skirts, shorts, and trousers for your body shape as discussed in the coming section: 'Styling Tips for the Different Body Shapes to Create Balance'. For example, if the hemline of the jacket ends at the widest part of the hips, it will accentuate and make the hips appear bigger.
- Wearing the right neckline for your face shape and body shape will be more slimming than wearing the wrong one.
- Avoid details and lines over your problem areas, as it will draw the eyes to that area.
- Shoes with higher heels will give the illusion that you are taller and slimmer. It does not have to be uncomfortably high, 3-5 centimetres (1-2 inches) in height can do the trick.

Extremely slim women can soften the angles of their figure with fullness in the fabric by using flowery prints, details, and soft pleats. Never wear over-sized clothes though. It must be your true size and the fullness must come in the style of the garment. For example, puff sleeves, pleated trousers and skirts, round lapels and hemlines of the garment, scarfs, beautiful soft dresses with A-line bottoms, white or light- and bright-coloured fabrics, which will all give the illusion of fullness and softness.

Styling Tips for the Different Body Shapes to Create Balance

Rectangle Body Shape

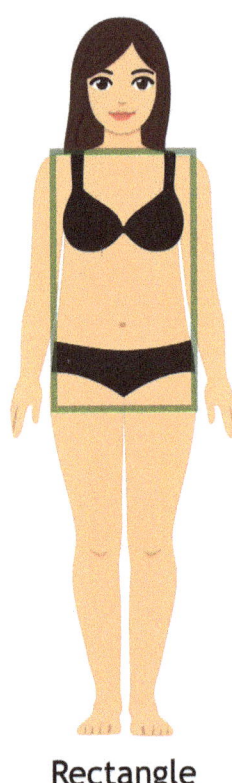

Rectangle

This body shape has straight lines and needs to be broken by adding curves and softness.

Shoulder pads will give extra width at the shoulders and the illusion of a smaller waist.

Wear lower, wider, scoop, and boat necklines, which will break the straight lines to provide curves.

Collars must be lifted and straight.

Sleeves can be a loose fit, puffed, cap, three-quarters in length, flared, cuffed or rolled up.

Jackets need to be structured with round lapels and/or necklines.

Asymmetric lines will create interest and draw the eyes away from the straight figure lines.

The younger and slimmer the figure, the shorter the skirt or dress can be, but not too short. Please do not just cover the bud because it will take away any elegance in the style.

Wear crossover, flip, panelled, or A-line skirts. Wear wide or bootleg pants, (no pockets); skinny jeans and trousers with beautiful tops.

Avoid any straight-line styles following the silhouette of the figure.

Avoid details at the waist, such as noticeable waistbands, belted jackets.

Avoid square and double-breasted jackets or coats as well as square pleats.

Opt for low- to medium-waisted trousers, that are straight and with a slight flare at the seam lines.

Avoid rectangle-shaped bags.

> The rectangle body shape appears square with straight side lines. The shoulder line, waistline, and hip line are basically the same width. The aim with all clothing styles should be to create curves with the illusion of a definite waistline. The shoulder line of jackets and tops needs to be wider than the actual shoulder width that will give an illusion of wider shoulders and, in effect, create balance.

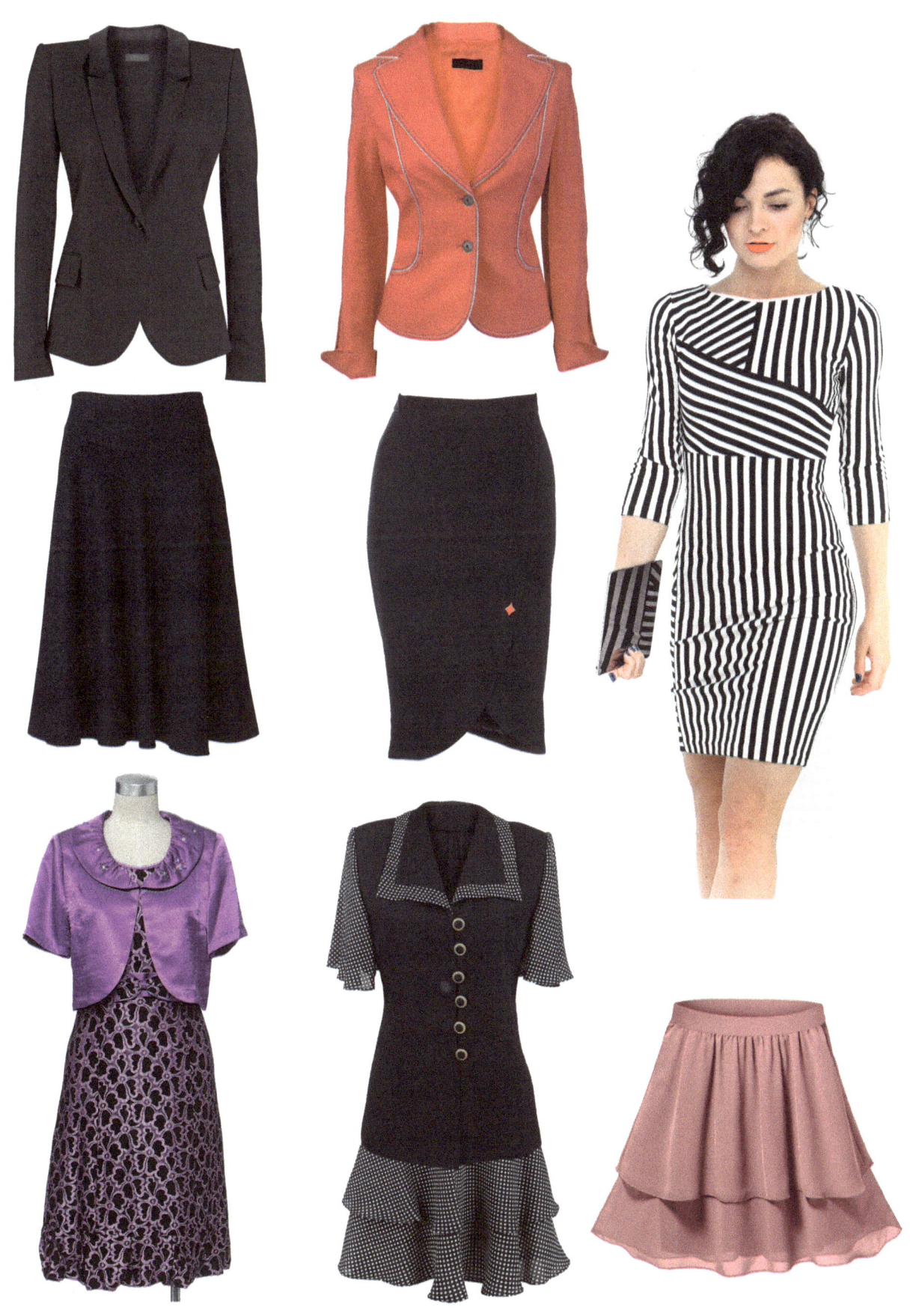

Style ideas for the rectangle body shape.

Inverted Triangle or Heart Body Shape

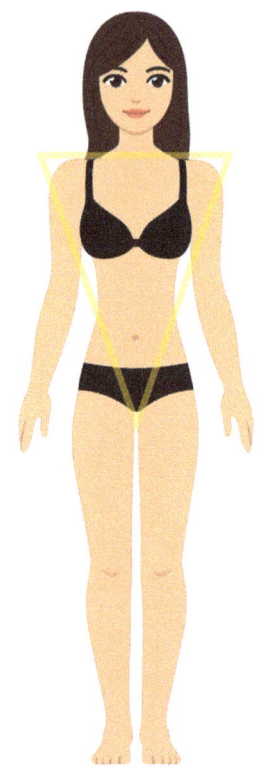

Inverted Triangle

The raglan sleeve will soften and camouflage wide arms.

Wear designs that bring the eye to the centre, such as the V-neckline or round neckline.

Avoid necklines that make you look broader, such as the boat or halter-neck.

Keep details and anything that creates volume to your lower half, and keep the top half clean and uncluttered.

Create the illusion of a waist with details such as a wider belt.

Vertical lines on the bodice will make the shoulders appear narrower.

High yokes with gathers and draped bodices help to visually reduce the full bust.

Avoid shoulder pads because it will extend the shoulders.

Avoid fabrics that cling to the body; wear fabrics that drape.

Avoid petite footwear because it will draw attention to the heavy upper half.

The inverted triangle body shape has a wider shoulder line with small hip, and the heart body shape has large boobs with small hips. Therefore, clothing styles must give the illusion of being smaller at the top and wider at the hips/bottom to create balance. The heart body shape is seen as sexy, and if the lady does not feel uncomfortable, she doesn't need to make her top look smaller. Be mindful of a too-low neckline. Too much of breasts exposure comes across as unprofessional.

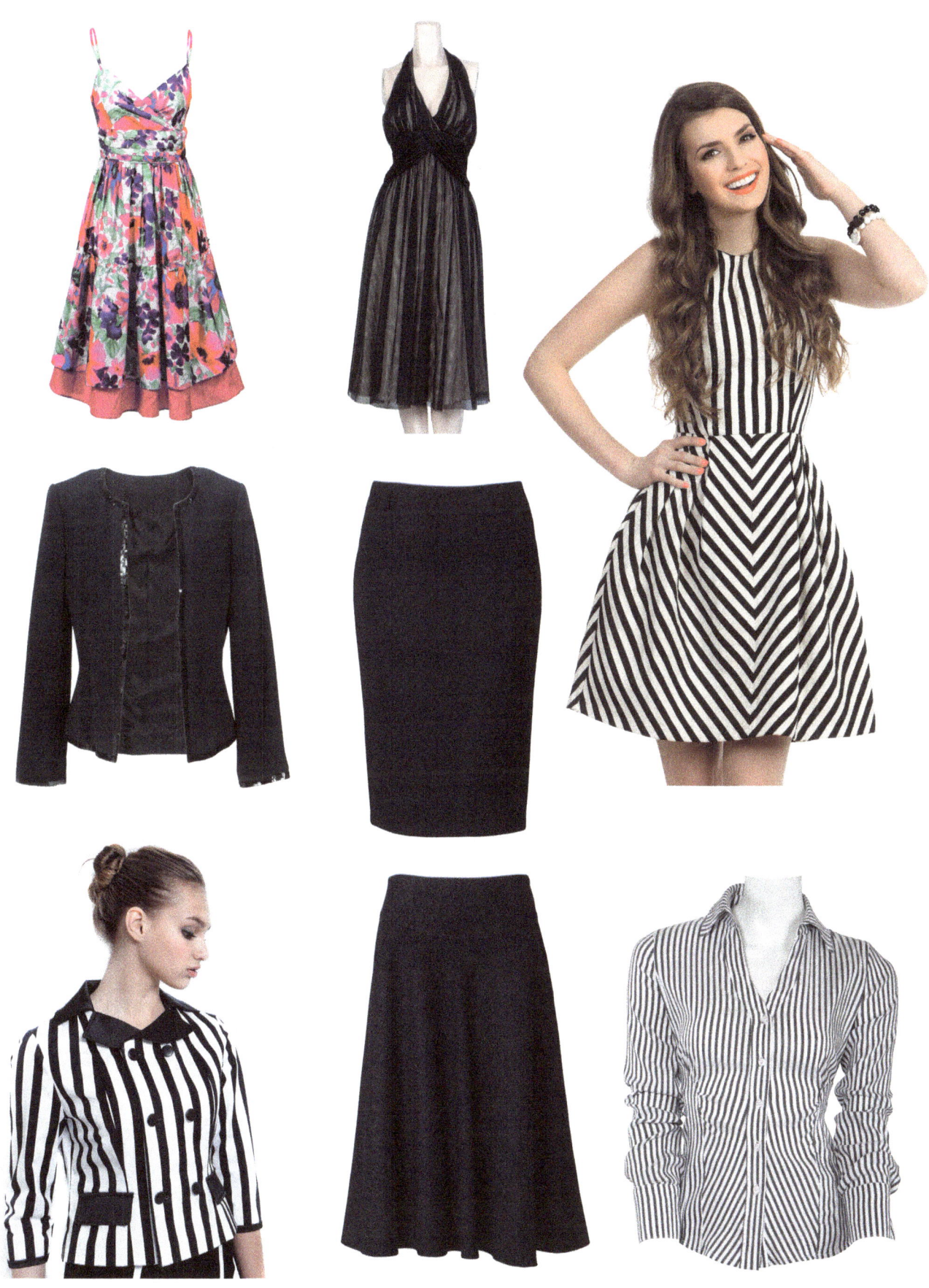

Style ideas for the inverted triangle or heart body shape.

Hourglass Body Shape

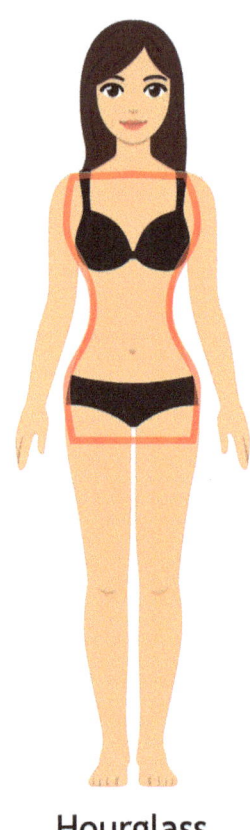

Hourglass

This is the most classic feminine shape, and women with this body shape can wear just about anything.

Shoulder pads will straighten and extend the shoulders past the thickest part of arms and hips and create the perfect balance of the shoulders being slightly wider than the hips.

Wear soft, curvy styles that follow the silhouette.

Straight-cut skirts or flowing. A-frame skirts is ideal.

Details at the shoulders, waist, and hemline will look great.

Avoid outfits that are too clingy or tight because it will add visual weight.

Skirts of any length will work, but be careful of very short skirts, as it can throw the perfect body shape off balance.

Avoid tight fabrics below the waistline because it will change the perfect balance you already have by making your bottom part appear much smaller than the shoulder line.

The hourglass body shape has a perfect balance where the shoulder line and hip line are the same width or have a very small difference of 3 centimetres. There is a definite waistline. Because of the perfect balance, this body shape can wear almost anything depending on the height of the lady. Shorter hourglass figures must also read the petite body shape style recommendations to give them the illusion of height.

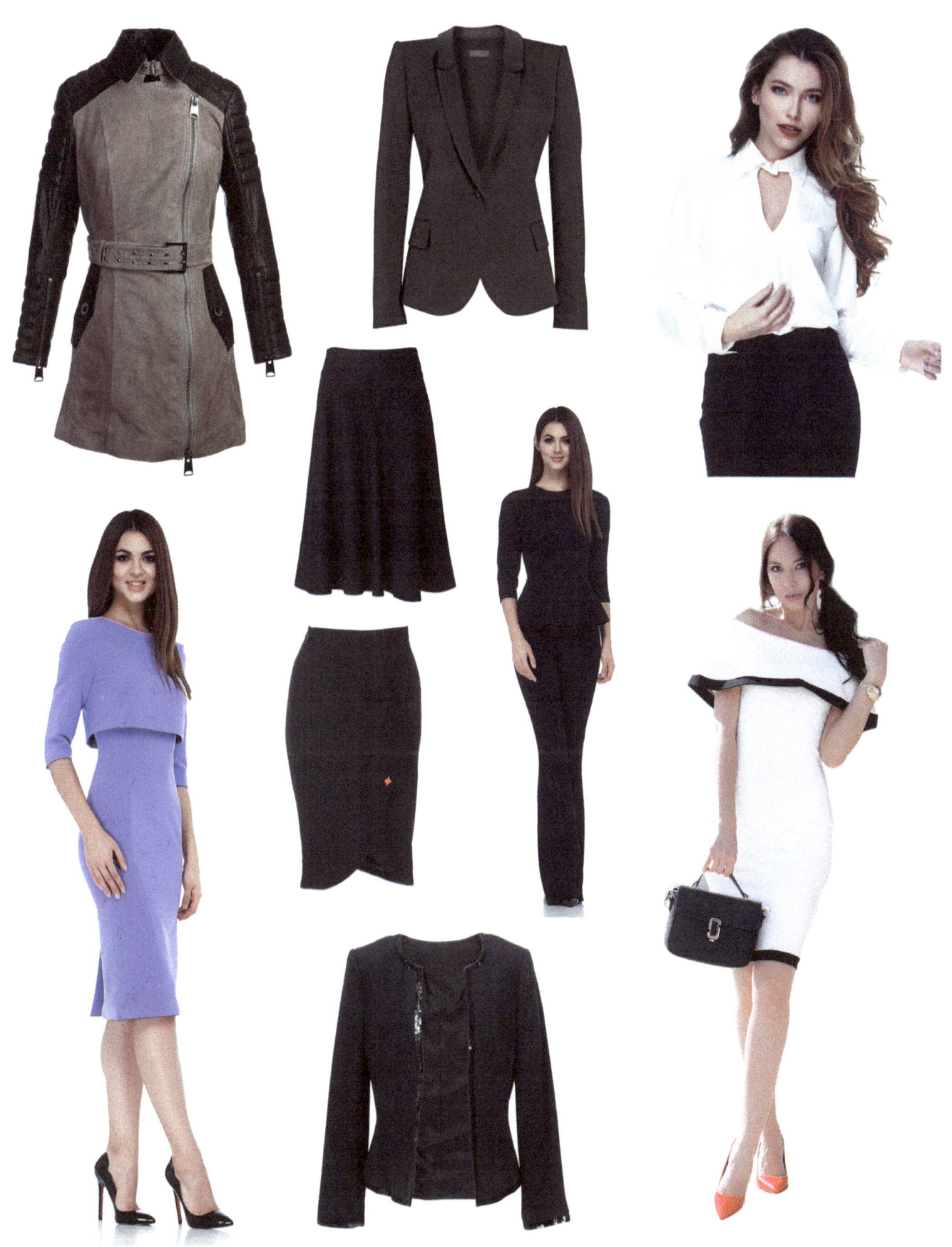

Style ideas for the hourglass body shape.

Round/Apple Body Shape

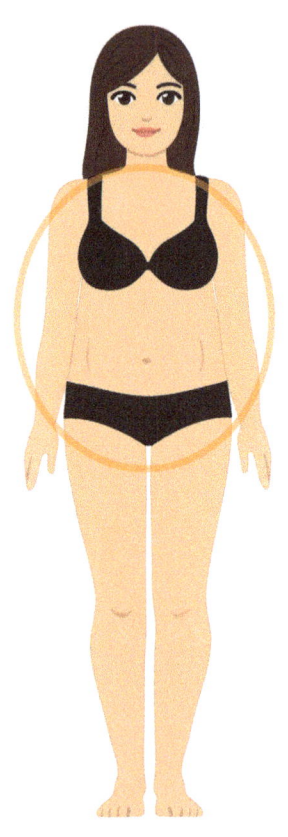

Round/Apple

Shoulder pads will make the shoulders look broader and clothes will drape well.

Wear long, straight-tapered jackets with tapered knee length skirts.

The best style of dresses will fall from the shoulder and taper towards the hem at the knee.

Keep details above the bust-line (collars and large jewellery), and below the hip line.

Avoid details and volume near the bust, tummy, or hips.

A short neck can wear low necklines, and a long neck, high necklines.

Wear vertical and diagonal lines in the fabric prints and designs that have a slimming illusion.

Avoid horizontal lines, which will add width.

Avoid jackets and cardigans finishing at your fullest body parts.

Avoid lapels, double-breasted coats or jackets, high-waisted trousers, belts or waistbands that will add fullness or draw attention to the widest body parts.

Avoid petite shoes, too thin high heels, boots with buckles, and UGG-boots. They will make you appear shorter and fuller.

> The round/apple body shape is widest at the middle and waist area. The shoulder line is usually much smaller. Clothing styles should create the illusion of a wider shoulder line and smaller tummy/middle area. This body shape will appear shorter because of the wide middle area. By wearing vertical lines and A-line designs with a waistband around the smallest part of the chest area (below the boobs), should give the illusion of being smaller. Asymmetrical designs are a great choice, which will create interest, and draw the eyes away from the fullness.

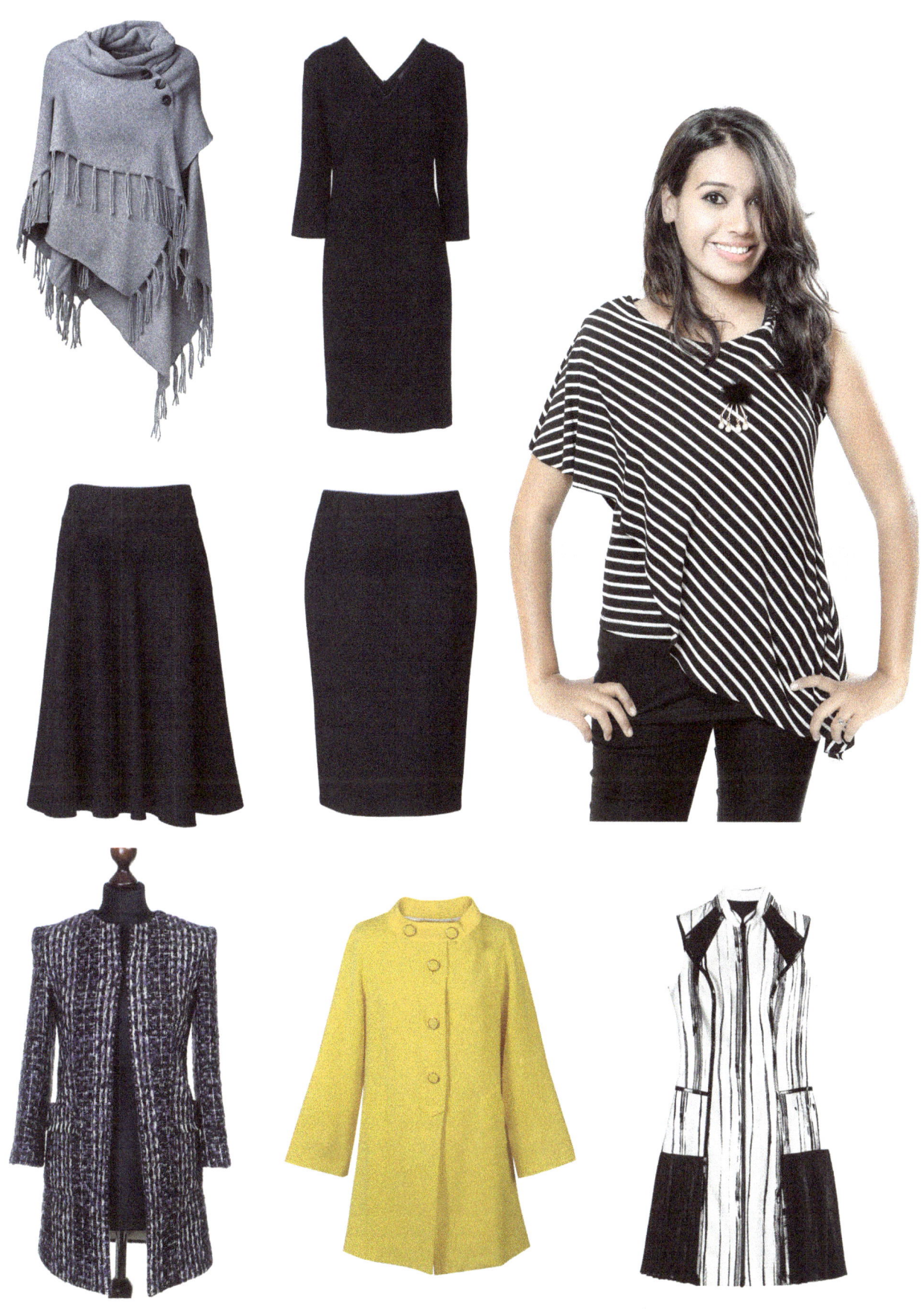

Style ideas for the round/apple body shape.

Triangle/Pear Body Shape

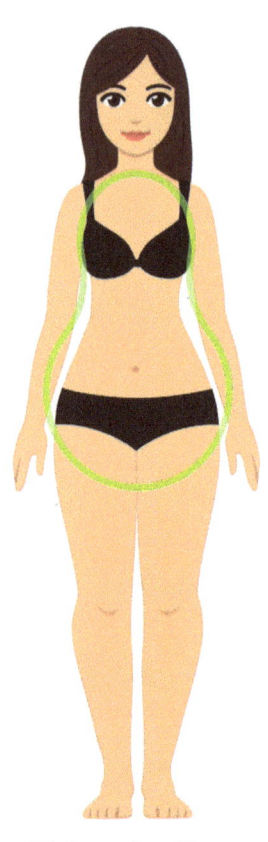

Triangle/Pear

Make your shoulders look broader with shoulder pads, puffed sleeves, cap sleeves, raglan shoulder lines, and boleros (short open jackets).

Jackets and tops need to finish above or below the hips and bottom.

Wear horizontal lines on the bodice to create width.

Wear vertical lines, diagonal lines, asymmetric styles, or darker one-colour skirts or trousers that will minimize the broad hips and bottom.

Wear straight-tapered knee-length skirts.

Curved and horizontal lines can be worn on the upper body.

Large straight collars will create a better balance between the top half and bottom half of the body, than shirts with no collars.

Scarves will work well to balance the top half with the larger hips and bottom.

Avoid miniskirts or any hemline of jackets finishing on the hips and thighs.

Avoid details, patterns, and pockets on the thigh, hip, and bottom area, which will create extra fullness and width.

Avoid horizontal lines on the bottom half. Rather, wear darker or one-colour fabric skirts and trousers, which will minimize the heavy bottom.

The triangle/pear body shape has a large bottom and hips, and narrow and small shoulders. To create balance, you'll have to make the shoulders appear wider and the hips and bottom appear smaller. The large bottom can also make this body shape appear shorter. To give the illusion of height, wear beautiful large and straight collars, vertical lines in the print or pattern of the lower body, and healthy high-heeled shoes.

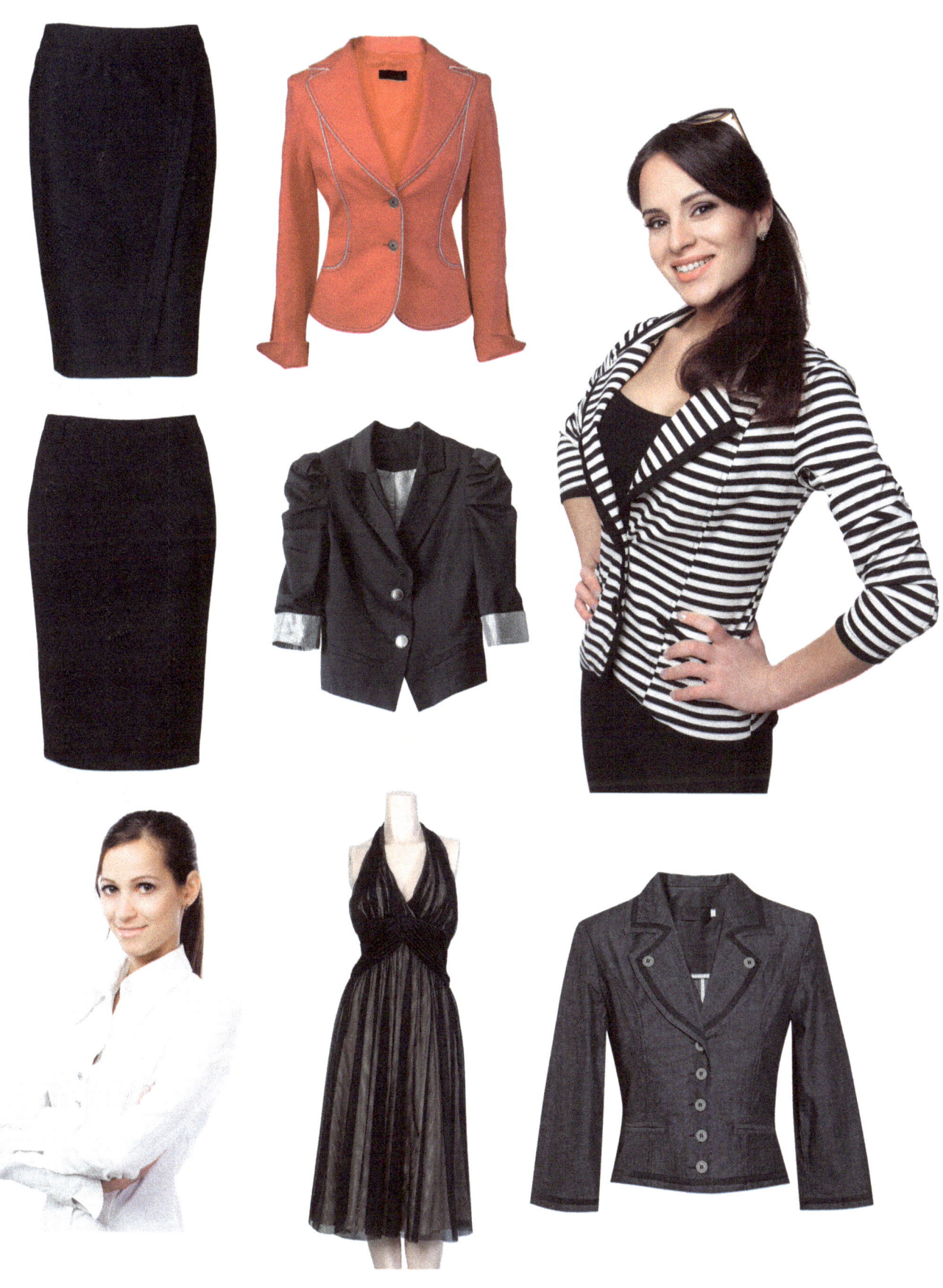

Style ideas for the triangle/pear body shape.

Petite Body Shape

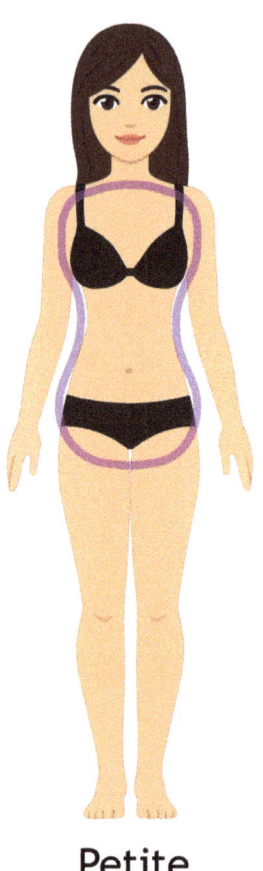

Petite

The petite is shorter than 158 centimetres and can be any of the already mentioned body shapes. The overweight petite can also follow the below tips but should not wear too-tight clothes.

Wear small medium-sized shoulder pads which will extend and make the shoulders look straight and a bit broader than the hips, which also adds height.

Wear straight yokes and collars, and wide lapels, which will draw the eyes up and give the illusion of extra height.

Wear straight-tapered knee-length skirts.

Avoid horizontal lines and stick with vertical and diagonal lines that give the illusion of length.

Jackets can stop at the waistline with small shoulder pads or have a cutaway hemline to give the illusion of height.

Small-sized belts in the same colour as the garment will work best for the fuller figure and small- to medium-sized belts for the slimmer figure.

Avoid pleats around the hips and wide waistbands, which will divide the figure and make it appear shorter.

> The petite body shape is short and will need to create the illusion of overall height. Create height at the shoulder area through small to medium-sized shoulder pads, straight collars, vertical lines, straight-cut patterns rather than frilly and A-line designs. Wear healthy high-heeled shoes and smaller accessories, like handbags, jewellery, and scarfs.

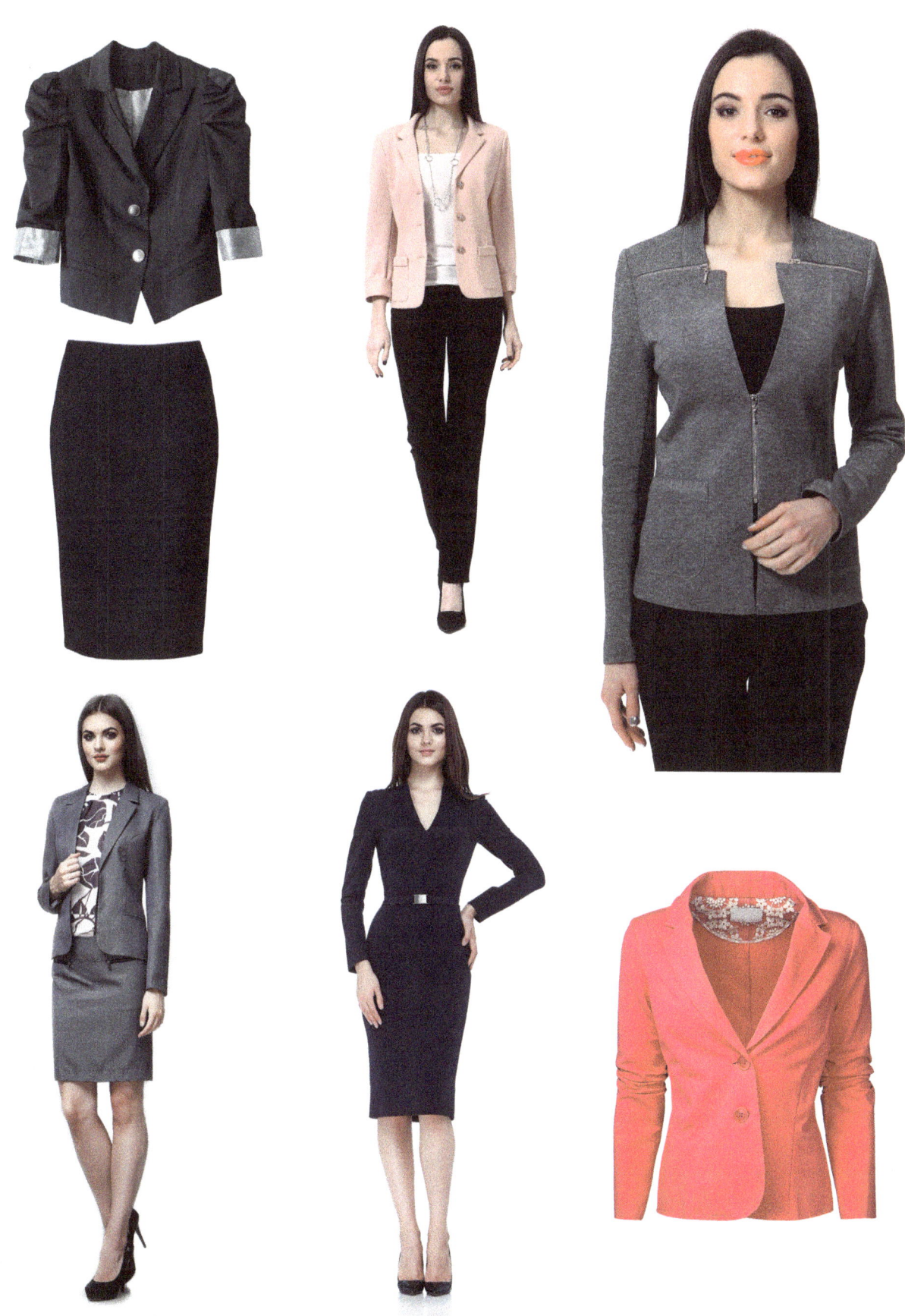

Style ideas for the petite body shape.

Lean Body Shape

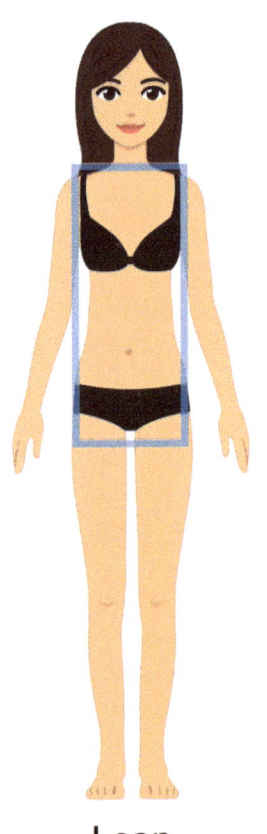

Lean

Shoulder pads will give extra width at the shoulders and the illusion of a waist.

Opt for lower, wider, scoop, and boat necklines.

Collars need to be straight.

Loose-fitted, puffed, cap, three-quarter, flared, cuffed or rolled-up sleeves will provide the needed curves this lean figure desperately needs.

Jackets need to be structured with round lapels and round necklines to break any hard lines the figure may project.

The lean figure can wear a shorter skirt or dress, but avoid too-short skirts which will expose bony legs. A-frame skirts and dresses with soft pleats (not square flat pleats), will add volume to the narrow hips.

Wear crossover, flip, panelled, and A-line skirts to create curves and more fullness.

Opt for low- to medium-waisted trousers, that are straight and with a slight flare.

Avoid details at the waist, such as noticeable waistbands, belted jackets.

Avoid square and double-breasted jackets or coats.

Avoid vertical lines that will draw attention to the lean silhouette, wear horizontal lines instead.

Avoid rectangle-shaped bags, and rather wear ovals and curved edges to soften the angular corners for the figure.

> The lean body shape is very lean with straight lines. Have no bust area, and may or may not have a waistline. You'll want to create overall fullness and curves with soft fabrics and pleats which will hide any hard lines. Wear light and pastel colours rather than black and darker colours, which give the illusion of being smaller. Colourful and large flowery dress fabrics should give some softness to the figure.

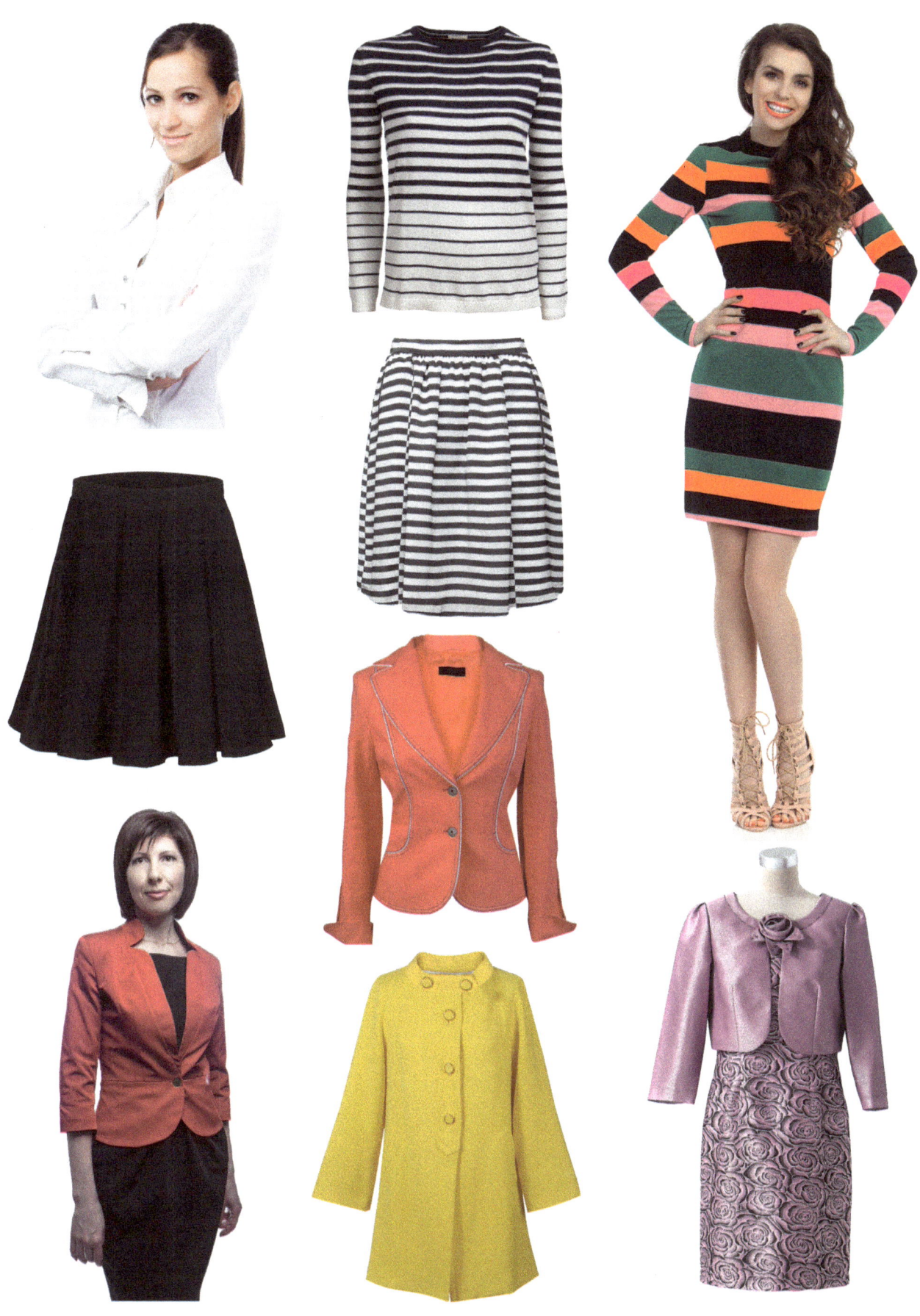

Style ideas for the lean body shape.

Plus-Size Body Shape

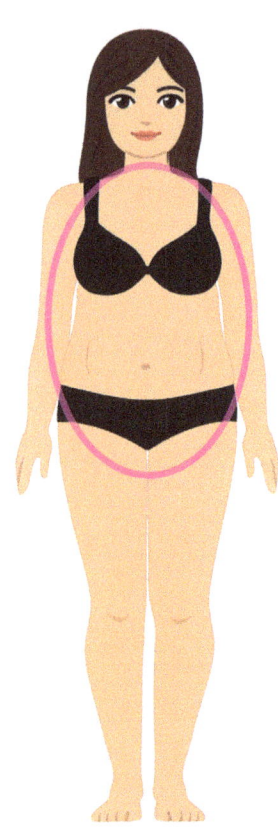

Plus Size

You can't go wrong with an A-line cut in a skirt. Avoid pencil skirts, as this shape will outline your hips and waist.

Do not wear oversized clothes, which will make you appear larger.

Wear vertical and diagonal lines, which will give a more slimming illusion.

Wear your underwear well-fitted. Good support will give shape and give the illusion of being smaller.

Choose tailored skirts and trousers.

The V-neckline is the most slimming for you.

Wear shirts with straight collars and short necklaces.

Wear a beautiful hairstyle, make-up, and earrings to draw the eyes up to your beautiful face.

The best shirts are tailored or soft and colourful with interesting fabric prints.

The set-in and raglan sleeve line is the most slimming.

Avoid horizontal lines and gathered fabrics that give the illusion of being larger.

Avoid flared- and wide-leg trousers.

Avoid leggings with short shirts. Thicker fabrics for trousers and jeans give more shape and are more slimming.

Avoid boleros (short cropped jackets), rather, wear full-length jackets with set-in sleeves and cardigans.

The plus-size body shape will want to give the illusion of being smaller and taller. This can be achieved through wearing tailored skirts, trousers, jackets, good support underwear, vertical lines, and V-necklines. This body shape is wider at the middle area and can give the illusion of being shorter. Vertical lines and tailored clothing designs will add height and have a slimming effect. Avoid any pleats and layers of fabric, which will create fullness.

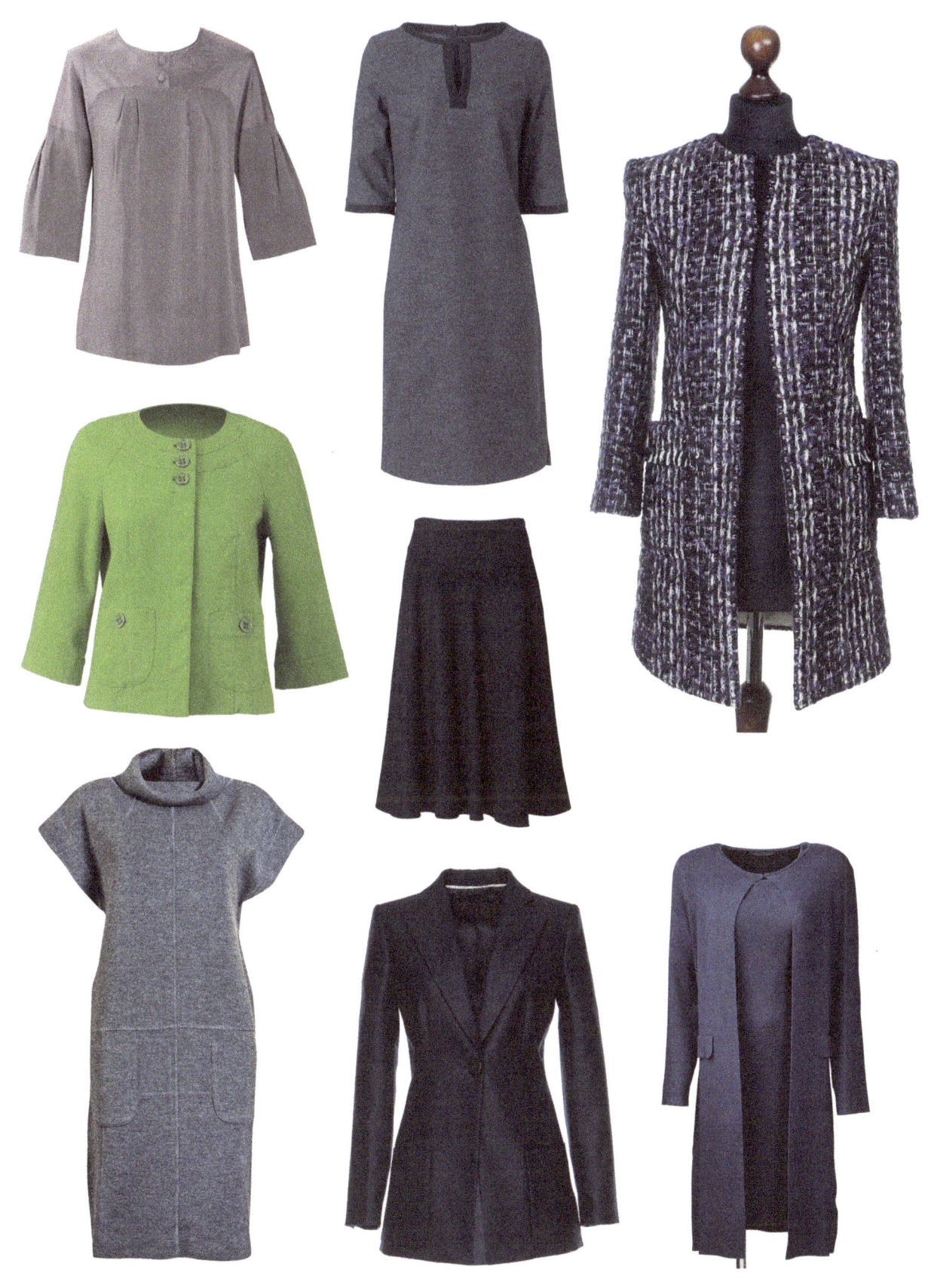

Style ideas for the plus-size body shape.

Choosing the Right Shoes

How to Choose Your Shoes

Buying high heels or flats? What is the best height of heels to wear? These are the questions on most women's mind. Some buy shoes because of the fashion, and others buy it only for comfort. I believe these two statements are both important, and we have to find the middle ground. Too-high and uncomfortable shoes can be detrimental to your health and posture, but flat shoes can also have a negative impact.

Your lifestyle, age, and type of work play the deciding factor when choosing the type of shoes you require. All women have a special occasion happening in their life every now and then where they want to look amazing. It does not look quite right when a woman wears a killer outfit and then finishes it off with flats. Shoes can be used as a finishing touch to any outfit. If you are 6 feet tall, you obviously would not want to wear high heels, but even heels that are 1-2 centimetres high will be better for foot health than flat soles. Let's compare it with women's running shoes. You do not get flat insole runners, they usually have an arch and thicker sole, which supports the foot better when running.

Not all shoe manufacturers have comfort and support in mind when they design shoes. When you are at home most of the day or walk long distances during the day, you will need comfortable shoes with great arch support. You have to do your research before stepping out to buy a new pair of shoes. Shoes must be so comfortable that you do not even realize you have it on for hours, even if they're high heels. Have you had a pair of shoes which was so comfortable that you wished you got more pairs of it than one? When you find a shoe style and brand that works well for you, try to stick with it.

You'll also find that price has nothing to do when it comes to comfort and support. What I want to bring across to you is, do not think that a thousand-dollar pair of shoes is going to last longer and is more comfortable than a hundred-dollar pair of shoes. The worst thing you can do for your health and posture is to wear shoes that cause any kind of pain and blisters while walking with them.

I have heard that some women believe by wearing bigger shoes than their foot size, they will avoid blisters. This is a wrong statement because on the other hand, it will create other nasty problems, such as muscles on the bottom of the foot that will tighten with each step in an attempt to keep the arch up. Shoes that is too big for you will bend in the wrong place and put stress on the wrong parts of the foot.

You will also notice that narrow shoes and very high heels are generally to blame for foot pain and lower back pain. Shoes that support the feet well allow the muscles of the foot to work less and ultimately lead to more comfortable shoes and less foot pain. Medical experts advise to avoid extremes, such as too-high heels or too-low heels.

Here are a few important tips when you buy shoes:

- A quick and easy way to determine which shoes will fit you is to stand on a piece of paper and trace your foot. Take the piece of paper with you when you are buying shoes. Place the shoes on top of the tracing first to see if it has the same shape and length of your foot.

- If it is too narrow or too short, do not even bother to fit it on. The upper part of the shoe should be in a soft fabric, such as leather, which is flexible and easily adjusts to the shape of your feet. The shape of the shoe should match the shape of your foot; if not, the shoe will be uncomfortable.
- The best time to buy shoes is in the afternoon when your feet has naturally expanded due to walking during the day.
- The toe region should be deep and roomy, allowing at least a 1-1.5 centimetres between your longest toe and the inside of the point of the shoe. Shoes that fasten to and around the foot with a buckle belt, strap, elastic, or laces will provide good support so that the shoes do not slip off when you're walking.
- The shoe should only bend where the foot bends, especially at the joint of the big toe.
- The heels of the shoes must fit snugly around your heel and not pinch or slip off. Fit both shoes, stand up, and walk around with them to make sure it fits well and is comfortable enough.
- Shoes should provide cushioning on the inside for the ball of each foot, which will prevent a burning ball when you walk and stand. The shoes shouldn't twist easily and must have good, sturdy support. The height of the heels must be in a healthy range for you and not too high.
- Never buy shoes purely for the look and fashion; comfort and support must come before fashion.
- Thin strapped sandals are not a good buy because the feet that balance and carry our body weight will not get the support they need.

Compare Heels

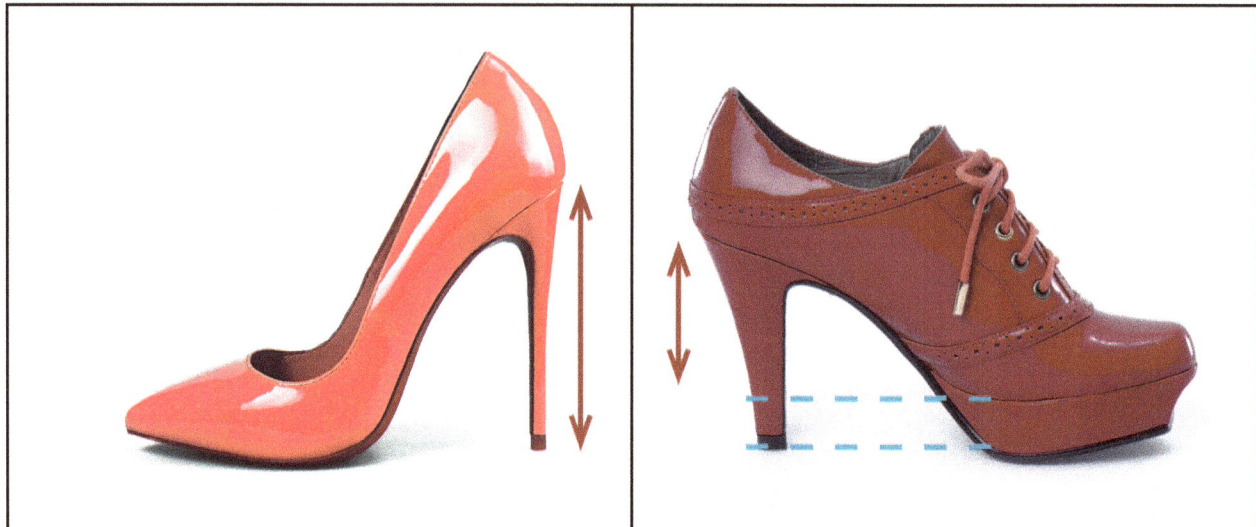

If you are a woman who really loves wearing heels, look at the above images of two different shoe styles. Look at the red shoe on the right and see how the thicker sole under the ball of the foot is cutting off some height from the heel. This shoe style with the thicker sole brings the actual height of the heel into a healthier range, and the thicker heel gives a more balanced grip to the ground or floor surface.

Now look at the coral-coloured shoe on the left. Can you see how the high heel forces the heel of the foot to be lifted? When the heel of the foot gets lifted to the maximum height, it will push the whole body's weight mainly to land on the ball of the foot. This unusual body posture again will be throwing the hips more forward, creating an unhealthy bend in the lower back. Even the knees will move more forward to keep the body balanced, putting extra stress on them. Try standing this way barefoot and lift your heels to the highest you can, then walk around for a few steps. Can you feel how unbalanced you are and the pain you most likely feel now on the balls of the feet, knees, and lower back? Although the high heel will give some support, the percentage will be very small.

The other question that gets asked often is this: can foot pain and unhealthy pressure really cause any other problems in the body?

Look at the following reflexology chart. The theory behind reflexology is that these areas correspond to organs and systems of the body. Proponents believe that pressure applied to these areas affects the organs and benefits the person's health; this includes practitioners of reflexology, such as chiropractors, physical therapists, massage therapists, and others. I believe that the wrong pressure and pain caused by our shoes on certain areas of the feet, can cause pain and problems in the body as shown on the reflexology chart.

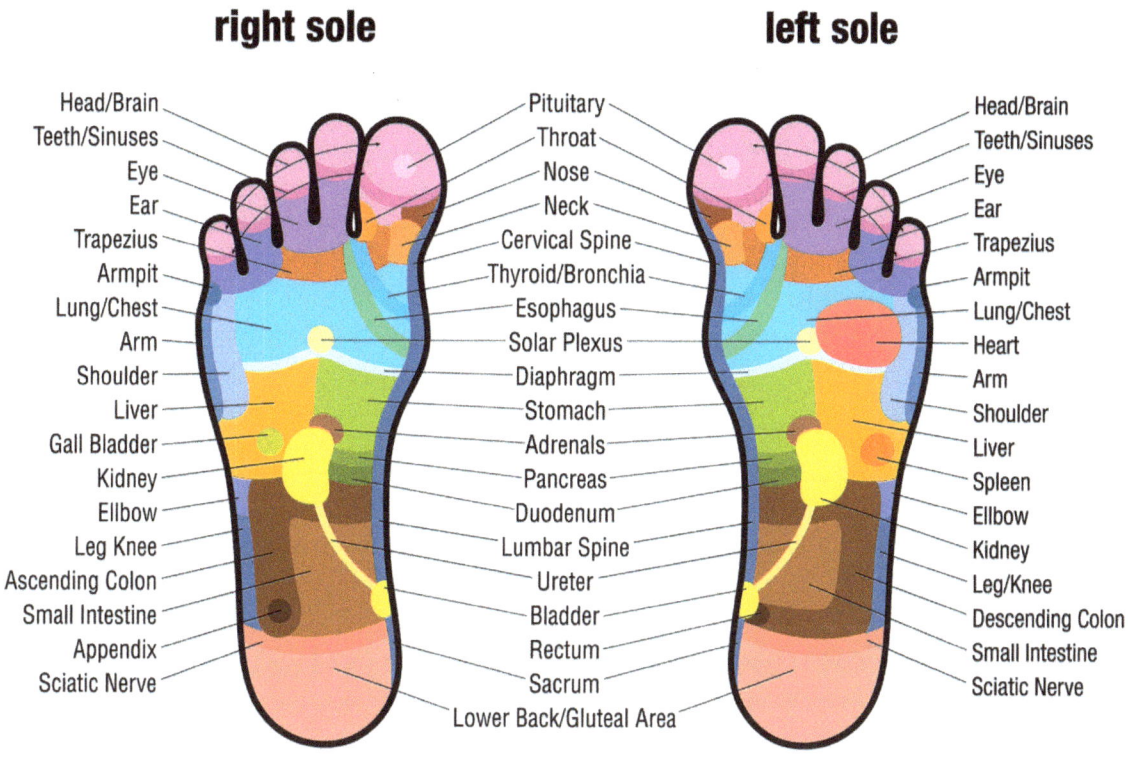

Reflexology chart.

The Main Reasons Why We Are Wearing Shoes

Shoes are to protect our feet and nails from any injury or germs coming from the outside world, such as the ground and floor surfaces. Injury can be caused by rocks, glass, sharp objects, or harmful liquids lying on the floor.

Certain shoes give a better grip to the surface you walk on and will allow you to walk faster or run faster than you would have barefoot.

The correct shoes will give your feet comfort and support. Your feet will feel warmer in winter or cold circumstances; good foot and ankle support will prevent any injuries to the muscles; enclosed shoes, like boots, will protect the feet from injuries coming from above, such as falling objects; a comfortable shoe fit will provide comfort for longer during the day.

Shoes with the right cushioning and style can correct your posture. For example, when you have a natural tendency to walk inwards with your feet, the right amount of build-up through cushioning inside of the shoe, can lift your feet and help you walk more straight.

This, again, will have a better impact on the rest of the body's alignments, ligaments, and posture.

Due to occupational health and safety standards, most organizations require that you wear the right shoes for a certain type of work to protect your feet from any injuries.

If we look outside work shoe requirements and think of our personal life when we go to meetings, interviews, special events, or outings, the shoe shape and style can improve the look of your outfit.

There are a few groups wondering why we need shoes and feel that our feet are created to form callouses, which should protect us when walking barefoot. I would say to those believers that they may enjoy a trip in Dr Brown's car (in the *Back to the Future* movie), to go back in time and enjoy walking barefoot. I for sure would not want hard, unsightly callouses on my feet. It does not matter what kind of work a woman does, she should always go back at night to look after herself through the right washing and grooming techniques. We are women, and we are beautiful! We have to do everything in our power to keep ourselves beautiful, not just for everyone around us, but mainly for ourselves. Looking well-groomed and beautiful will give us a boost of confidence.

How do you Clean Shoes

I had a young lady mentioned to me one day that her shoes really smell bad. I asked her if she wipes her shoes clean in the inside every now and then with a dampened cloth or cleaning wipe. She was quite embarrassed because she never thought to do that.

Just as everything that comes in contact with the sweat on our skin needs cleansing, shoes need wiping and cleaning on the inside as well. Our feet do sweat, especially in summertime and in the wintertime when we wear less-breathable shoes and socks to stay warm. A person does not have to be excessively hot to be excessively sweaty. Some women think that foot powder will get rid of the stinky problem, but in fact, it only helps to rid of the problem temporarily. Think about what will happen if we keep sprinkle carpet freshener on the carpet every time instead of vacuuming and cleaning it. There will be a build-up of powder and because of all the dirt and dust build-up as well, the carpet will get dirtier and start to smell badly.

The problem is that most do not realize that the contained sweat and warmth of the feet inside the shoes become a breeding ground for bacteria, which are the cause for the bad smell. These bacteria live on our feet, in our socks, and all over our shoes. If we do not clean the inside of our shoes regularly and wash our feet at least twice every day (morning and night), the bad smell will worsen. Another secret is to ventilate the feet during the day. I keep a pack of fragrance-free baby wipes that I buy at a low price from the supermarket in my handbag or car. When I feel my feet are sweaty, I'll wipe them and the inside of my shoes, each with their own wipe, to eliminate transferring bacteria from one to the other. If you use a dampened cloth, it is imperative to clean it before the next use. Only insert the feet back into the shoes when they have dried. To speed up the process, you can dry it quicker with tissue or toilet paper.

Eliminate Sweaty and Smelly Feet

Avoid shoes made of synthetic materials. Leather shoes are more breathable.

Wear a fresh pair of socks every day and never re-wear socks which have already been worn for a day.

Wash your feet daily, preferable twice daily (morning and night), and dry them thoroughly, especially between the toes, to eliminate any breeding ground for bacteria. On a long trip where you are not near a bath or shower, at least wipe your feet clean with cleaning wipes.

Make sure your feet are dried thoroughly as well before inserting them in enclosed shoes. You can spray your feet with an antiperspirant, which will keep your feet fresher for longer. Shoes with removable insoles can be cleaned easily by just removing them from the shoes to wash them; let them dry in the sun before placing them back in the shoes.

Alternate your shoes daily to allow them to dry thoroughly. Regularly wipe shoes clean inside and out.

Advice on How to Clean Leather and Synthetic Shoes

Outside

Use a soft dampened cloth to wipe the outside clean from any dirt or dust. Apply shoe polish, wax, or cream on the outside to help shine, and restore, and give waterproof protection to leather shoes. Ask the shoe boutique which product will be best to use for your shoes. They normally sell shoe-cleaning products in-store. You'll also find different shoe polishes in the supermarket, if you know what you are looking for.

After the polish dries, you can use a soft dry cloth to give it a shine. Most synthetic shoes and shoes with a glossy shine will not require any polish, and the best you can do is to wipe them clean with a dampened cloth and shine them with a soft dry cloth.

Inside

Use a dampened cloth with a bit of liquid hand soap or dishwashing liquid to wipe the inside clean, followed up by a dampened cloth with no soap to get rid of all the remaining soap in the shoe. Then dry it with a soft dry cloth.

Instead of a dampened cloth, you can use a normal or antibacterial wipe to sweep the inside of the shoes, followed by drying them with a piece of toilet paper or paper towel.

To deodorize the shoes, pour two tablespoons of baking soda into each shoe and shake the shoes to spread it out evenly. Be careful not to use baking soda on leather shoes. Let the shoes sit overnight, then shake and wipe the excess powder out, before wearing them.

Alternatively, you can use shoe powder.

Sneakers and Runners

There can be cleaning instructions on a label inside the sneaker/runner and most likely on the inside of the tongue part of the shoe. It can also be in the form of instructions inside the shoe box when you buy it. If you are not sure, ask the store salesperson about the best method to clean it. My preference is to buy sneakers and runners that will clean easy and will not collect or show dirt easily. For example, sneakers or runners in white fabric are something I will never buy since it is too hard to keep them looking like new and clean. To put sneakers and runners through the washing machine and tumble drier is not the right way. The water and the heat over a long wash cycle will break down the glues used in making it and will greatly reduce their lifespan.

The first step is to brush off all dirt, grass, and dust from the sneakers or runners with a soft, clean, and dry brush or shoe brush.

Remove any insoles and laces, and wash them separately with laundry liquid or a laundry bar of soap in the laundry tub. After the first wash, rinse them in clean water to remove most soap. Hang or place them in the sun to dry quickly. Replace any broken and old laces to give the sneakers/runners a newer look.

Fill a plastic laundry wash-tub or laundry tub with lukewarm water to about 2 centimetres, or where the water level reaches the halfway mark of the sneaker/runner's sole. Use an old nail brush and soap (laundry bar of soap or laundry powder) to brush the plastic soles clean. Do one sneaker/runner at a time and place it in another dry plastic tub or on a spot that you do not have to clean afterwards.

For a solid leather or synthetic leather top, clean with a dampened cloth only and very little liquid laundry soap. Do both sneakers and runners before rinsing all the soap out of the cloth. Finish off by wiping any remaining soap from the sneakers/runners. Place them outside to dry.

For a fabric top, use a sneaker/runner cleaner, which is almost like a shampoo, and a brush or cloth to brush and wipe them clean. Read the instructions for the specific cleaner that you use. What I do if my sneakers/runners cleaner is finished: I use a light carpet- or upholstery cleaner, using a sponge and cleaning with the foam. Be careful of too-strong cleaners though, which can affect the colour/s of the sneakers. Wipe and clean the insides as well. Leave the sneakers/runners outside to dry.

Only a minority of sneakers can be successfully submerged in water to wash. As soon as the insoles, laces, and sneakers/runners are dry, put them all together. With all the above cleaning techniques, you'll have beautiful, clean and fresher sneakers/runners; and with regular cleaning you will stretch its lifespan.

Walking in High Heels

High-Heeled Shoes

If you were never able to balance yourself on high-heeled shoes before, it is because your ankle muscles and calf muscles are not strong enough. You can strengthen the muscles so that it would be easier to walk with high heels. Just a friendly reminder: I do not mean unhealthy high heels but those between 3-5 centimetres (1-2 inches) high, that still fall in the healthier range.

Wearing heels will lift your ankles and put the calf muscles in a shortened position. That is why you will experience pain in your ankles or knees. By stretching and strengthening the muscles in the ankles and lower legs regularly, you will combat any pain or accidents when walking with high heels.

Do the Following Foot, Ankle, and Calf Muscle Exercises

1. Stand behind a chair, and let your hands help you balance on the back of the chair. Raise your heels so you are standing on your toes, and then set your feet back down. Repeat this exercise for ten to fifteen times.

2. Stand on one leg at a time and balance for fifteen seconds. Keep the chair in front of you for in case you have to keep yourself from falling. Once that gets easy, increase the time.

3. Lift the front part of your feet off the floor and balance on your heels while walking as far as you can in the room and, if possible, across the whole room. Repeat a couple of times.

4. Raise your heels and walk on the ball of your feet across the room. Repeat a couple of times.

5. Jumping rope is a great exercise to strengthen ligaments and ankle muscles.

6. Use a small hard ball, such as a tennis or golf ball. Stand near a wall to help you keep your balance. Now place the ball under the arch of one foot and roll the ball up and down your foot for one minute. You can control the intensity by shifting your weight. Repeat this exercise with the other foot.

7. Sit on a chair with your back straight. Now cross your right ankle over the left knee so that the foot hangs free. Draw the entire alphabet with your big toe. Once all twenty-six letters are completed, switch legs and repeat this exercise.

How Can You Look Natural When Walking with High Heels?

First, make sure that the heels you are wearing are not too high. When you walk, put your heel down first, followed by a rolling movement from the ball of your foot to the toe. Then push yourself slightly forward for the next step.

How Do You Get Used to Wearing High Heels if You've Always Worn Flats?

Do your foot, ankle, and calf muscle exercises regularly, and walk for short periods of time with your high heels. For example, walk for five minutes at a time, and when it does not feel that uncomfortable any more, increase to ten and later to fifteen minutes. Keep increasing the time that you are walking with the high heels until you can walk for five to eight hours during the day. Swap with comfortable shoes that have a slight heel of 1-2 centimetres to wear in between times.

Why Are Flat Shoes Bad for You?

The lack of arch support and cushioning in flat shoes can actually damage your feet. The most common causes of foot pain are fallen arches, also known as flat feet, which are normally a genetic condition but can be aggravated by footwear without any arch support. When the arch in the foot drops, the ligaments and tendons in the base of the foot will overstretch and cause continuous pain.

If you really want to wear flats, make sure they have enough arch support, and avoid flat shoes with thin soles.

Flat shoes can also cause plantar fasciitis. This is a condition where the fascia ligament of the foot gets inflamed as a result of strain injury, that is caused by micro tears in the ligament as it attaches to the heel bone or other areas of tightness on the sole of the foot. Plantar fasciitis is most commonly caused by repetitive strain injury to the ligament of the sole of the foot. Excessive running, walking, or jumping in shoes with inadequate arch support, can cause plantar fasciitis, but can also be caused by certain diseases. The main symptoms of plantar fasciitis are heel pain, foot pain, tenderness, stiffness. In the case where you have really bad foot pain constantly, it is always good to see your physician to make sure there is nothing to worry about.

Find Your Colours

Find Your Perfect Colours to Wear

There is no use in finding your perfect style through this book and not knowing your best colours to wear. Colour is extremely important when it comes to getting dressed. It is very much like make-up and hairstyles that flatter your skin tone and face shape. The correct colours and style can complement your overall skin tone and body shape. If you get the colours wrong, it can make you look tired and even ill. The wrong colours often depreciate you where people see your clothes before they see you. We want people to notice us as a person first, rather than noticing our clothes. One of the compliments we get when people notice us is when they say 'You look beautiful today!', and not 'You have a beautiful dress' or 'I like your dress'.

Some women spend thousands of dollars on style to get others to notice them. The good news is that you do not need to spend thousands on clothing to look amazing. When you have the colour and style that fit your skin tone, body shape, and personality, you will look a million dollars. There is also no shame if you spend good money on a designer outfit every now and then, if you have the budget for it.

Finding your right colours can do the following for you:

- It makes you *look* healthier, younger, slimmer, and brighter.
- It also makes you *feel* healthier, younger, slimmer, and brighter.
- Colour can affect your mood and emotions.
- Can help you create the illusion of the perfect and/or slimmer body shape.
- Your eyes, skin, and hair will glow when they are well-groomed as well.
- Imperfections such as dark eye circles and discoloration will be reduced, meaning that you need less make-up.
- You will appear smart and sharp.

With the wrong colours:

- Your eyes, skin, and hair will look dull and drained.
- Imperfections (such as a double-chin, dark eye circles, yellow teeth, etc.) will be highlighted and even created.
- Your face will fade into the background, while the colours will stand out.

Knowing all this, the question to ask is, why would you want to wear the wrong colours?

There are a wide variety of approaches to analysing personal colouring today. Carole Jackson wrote the book *Color Me Beautiful* in 1980, which had the world very excited about the correct colours to wear during the eighties and onwards. She simplified Caygill's seasonal system, that used sixteen different personalities per season, and reduced it to a single personality per season. Thanks to Carole Jackson's simplified theory, discovering your season became pretty straightforward, and women found it easier to discover their right colours. She named it after the four seasons and the colours found in nature to help remember the range of colours they include. The four colour season analysis consists of winter, summer, autumn, and spring.

More recently, a new personal colour analysis system has seen the light; it is called the flow colour analysis. This new system is based on the traditional four seasons from *Color Me Beautiful*, but takes into account that some women do not fall into one season only and can have features of another season.

When these four seasons flow into one another, it creates twelve new colour groups, also called the Flow Colour Analysis. They are as follows:

1. Light spring
2. Clear spring
3. Warm spring
4. Light summer
5. Soft summer
6. Cool summer
7. Deep autumn
8. Soft autumn
9. Warm autumn
10. Deep winter
11. Clear winter
12. Cool winter

These twelve categories are discussed in more detail after the four seasons are explained in the following pages.

The Factors Determining Skin Colour

The skin colour of each person is determined at birth, and is a part of his or her heritage that cannot be changed. There are three main pigments in the skin that gives you your unique skin colour: melanin, haemoglobin, and carotene. They are found in the dermis skin layer just underneath the outer skin layer that we can see and feel, called the epidermis. These three pigments combine to produce the pigmentation of all surface tissues, including the skin, mucous membranes, and even the eyes. Abnormal concentrations of these pigments can cause distinctive colour changes in the skin or other visible body tissues and may help in the diagnosis of certain illnesses or skin conditions.

Human skin colour ranges in variety from the darkest brown to the lightest hues. A person's skin colour is the result of genetics, and the product of both biological parents' genetic make-up.

Melanin is produced within the skin cells called melanocytes, and it is the main determinant of the skin colour of darker-skinned humans. The skin colour of people with light skin is determined mainly by the bluish-white connective tissue under the dermis and by the haemoglobin circulating in the veins of the dermis. The red colour underlying the skin becomes more visible, especially in the face, when capillaries on the surface dilate as consequence of physical exercise or the stimulation of the nervous system when angry and fearful. Colour is not entirely uniform across an individual's skin; for example, the skin of the palm and the sole is lighter than most other skin, and this is especially noticeable in darker-skinned people.

Melanin

Of all three pigments, melanin is the most powerful. The cells that produce it are the same in all races, but there is wide variation in the amount produced and its colour, ranging from black to light tan. Every adult has about 60,000 melanin-producing cells in each square inch of skin. Melanin cells also affect eye colour. When the cells are deep in the eye, the colour produced is blue or green. When they are close to the surface, the eye is brown. Albinism is a disorder where there is no melanin present and the eyes will appear pink, because the stronger pigment that ordinarily masks the blood vessels is lacking.

Haemoglobin

The pigment that gives blood its colour is called haemoglobin and has the second greatest effect on skin colour. When it combines with oxygen, a bright red is the result, and this in turn produces the rosy complexion associated with good health in light-skinned people. When such people suffer from reduced haemoglobin because of anaemia, they appear to be excessively pale. A concentration of reduced haemoglobin gives the skin a bluish appearance. Because haemoglobin has a weaker colouring effect than melanin, which determines basic skin colour, these variations are more visible in lighter-skinned individuals.

Carotenes

The weakest pigments in the skin are the carotenes. They produce a yellowish tone that is increased by eating excessive amounts of carrots and oranges. In people with darker skin, excess carotene is usually masked by the melanin pigment. Beta-carotene has an orange to yellow colour. There are reports that excessive intake of beta-carotene for a significant length of time may cause a yellow or orange discoloration of the skin. Commonly, this discoloration is found in the palms of the hands and soles of the feet. The sclera and membranes of the eyes, nose, and mouth are not discoloured by beta-carotene.

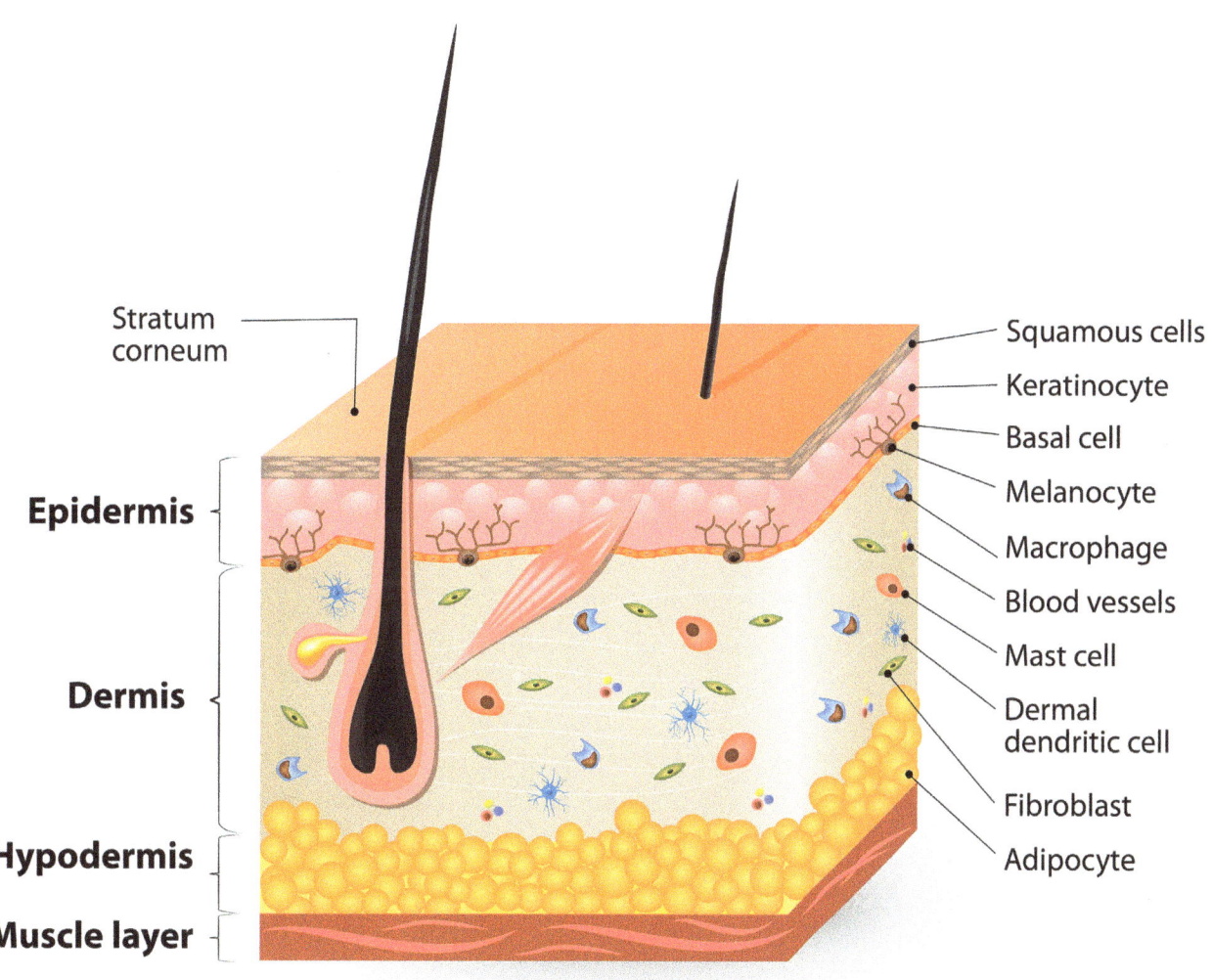

Illustration of the human skin.

Skin Undertone

There are many different shades of skin, but only two main undertones. The two tones are *cool* and *warm*. Turn your palms facing up, and look at the colour of the veins on your wrist. Blue or purple coloured veins will make you 'cool' toned. If they look green or have a yellow cast, you are 'warm' toned. Cool-toned women look best in what we call 'cool colours', such as white, black, royal blue, grey, navy. Think of colours that remind you of water, sea, and sky. Metallic and silver is your best fit. Warm tones look beautiful in earthy shades, like orange, cream, saturated sunny yellow, brown, dark leafy green, and that shade of red maple leaves turn into when autumn starts. When you are a mixed of blue/purple and green veins, you have a neutral undertone. Women with a neutral skin undertone can wear any colour on the colour wheel, but it's best to stick with the softened or muted colour versions, instead of the bright ones.

How to Determine Whether Your Skin Tone Is *Cool* or *Warm*

It involves looking beyond your skin colour and discovering the undertone that gives definition to your specific looks. Your skin tone is determined by the amount of melanin, or pigment, in your skin and does not change from sun exposure. Your skin tone will be one of the following: cool, warm, or neutral. Perform the following three tests to determine your skin under-tone. To make sure the tests are accurate, perform it in a room with natural light. Artificial light can influence the test. The piece of paper or fabric that you are going to use for test one, must be large enough to cover a good amount of skin. Drapes must cover both shoulders.

Test 1: Gold and Silver Test

Take one silver-coloured piece of fabric and a gold-coloured piece of fabric or paper. Place one hand on the silver-coloured piece and the other hand on the gold-coloured piece. Also try the inner side of your wrists or another part of your body that gets rare sun exposure. You will notice that with the right colour, your skin colour will blend in well with the colour of the paper or fabric, and your skin will look even. With the wrong colour, your skin will look uneven and speckled. You can even use dress fabric drapes in solid gold and solid silver to drape around your shoulders. Preform this test without any make-up on because it can give you the wrong results. Now see which drape makes your face glow.

Silver equals *cool*; and gold means *warm*.

Test 2: Foundation Test

Another accurate method involves putting a dab of pink-based cream foundation on one cheek, and a dab of yellow on the other. Then spread the foundation evenly on each cheek until they form a very thin layer. Finally, look at which one blends in versus which looks painted on. The one that blends better with you is your match.

Pink means *cool*; yellow means *warm*.

Test 3: Vein Test

Look at the veins on your inner wrist and determine whether they look more bluish or greenish. Make sure you conduct the test in natural light. Do not do this test right after tanning or if you have a deep tan, as it makes it more difficult to determine the colour.

Green veins mean *warm*; blue means *cool*.

If your veins are both blue and green, you have a *neutral* undertone. You can wear anything on the colour wheel, but it is best to go for softened or muted versions of a colour instead of the brighter ones.

Another easy test is to take a piece of white paper and hold it under your wrist and hand for comparison. Is your skin blue, blue-pink, golden, or even orange? If your skin is tanned, look at the part of your body that is not changed by the sun. What colour is your freckles, charcoal brown or golden brown? Charcoal means you are *cool*, and golden brown makes you *warm*.

Cool Undertone	Warm Undertone
You are a	You are a
summer or *winter*.	*spring* or *autumn*.

The Four Colour Seasons

Our skin tone is not always that obvious. The following are more-complete descriptions of the various types of colouring according to Carole Jackson's findings that typify each season, including hair and eyes.

Winter

The skin has a blue or blue-pink undertone and is classified as *cool*. Most olive- to dark-skinned women, Asians (including Chinese, Japanese, Korean), and European women are winters, although a few can be autumns. The skin colour of some winters can appear golden, that makes it difficult to determine the exact skin tone. When they wear golden colours the skin will appear pale, while cool winter colours bring them to life. A woman who is a winter may also have milky-white skin and dark hair like the portrait in the well-known children's story, *Snow White*. The white skin may have a visible pink tone or have a translucent quality and usually do not have rosy cheeks. Their appearance improves dramatically with pinkish tone blushers. There are more winters in the world than any other season type.

Eye colours are most often a deep colour, such as black–brown, dark blue, blue (with flecks in the iris and maybe a grey rim), dark red-brown, hazel, grey-blue, grey-green or green (with flecks in the iris and maybe a grey rim). Grey-rimmed eyes mean you are one of the 'cool' seasons, winter or summer.

Most winters have dark hair even when they were white-blonde in childhood. Blue-black hair is common of the winter colour season personality, and when they turn grey, it can be a salt-and-pepper or silver-grey colour. A brunette winter's hair colour ranges from light brown to dark charcoal brown, sometimes with a touch of red highlights. Of all the colour personalities, the winter is the most likely to grey prematurely, and often grey attractively. You'll rarely find a winter who is naturally blonde as an adult, but if she is, her hair is a white-blonde.

Summer

The skin has blue-colour veins, creating a *cool* undertone. They usually have visible pink in their skin. Some summers are very fair and may have a translucent quality to the skin. Other summers have very pink skin with deep rose-beige and a visible pink in the cheeks.

Eye colours are most often blue with brown flecks around the pupil, blue with white flecks in the iris and maybe a grey rim, grey-blue, clear bright blue, clear pale aqua (and changes from blue to green, depending on the colour of the shirt or bodice), grey-green, green with white flecks and maybe a grey rim, pale grey, hazel (blue and brown or green and brown), soft brown.

Hair colour is most often blonde to ash blonde. As the summer woman matures, the colour tends to darken and have a greyish cast. At times, a summer has auburn highlights in their hair, especially when she is often in the sun. Brunettes have hair colours ranging from light to dark brown, again with ash undertones. Summers grey gracefully to a blue-grey or pearly-white tone.

Autumn

Women who are an autumn colour season personality is more orange than blue, the golden undertone that classifies as *warm*. The autumn can fall in one of three categories: (*a*) the woman with ivory or creamy-peach skin; (*b*) the true redhead, who is fair to dark and often have freckles; (*c*) the brunette whose golden-beige skin can range from medium to deep copper and who has charcoal-black hair as she matures. Many autumns are pale with colourless cheeks, and an orange-toned blusher will make them look brighter. Autumns and springs have similar colouring, the only difference is that springs have rosy cheeks. A few Asians and Africans are autumns, if they have truly golden undertones.

Most autumns have brown or green eyes and can be any of the following variations: dark to golden browns, hazel (golden brown or green gold), amber, green with brown or golden flecks, pale to clear greens, blue with a distinct aqua or turquoise tone.

Many autumns are brunettes, and their hair usually have a gold or metallic red cast. Occasionally, an autumn has charcoal-black hair. They can be golden blonde as a child and usually darkens as they mature. Redheads' hair colour ranges from carrot orange to those with auburn or red-brown hair. A few redheads are springs because their colouring is too delicate to handle the stronger autumn palette.

Spring

Of all four colour season personalities, the spring has the most delicate quality and is the most likely to have rosy cheeks. Their skin is usually finely textured, and colour seems to rush to the surface quickly; they blush easily. Look for the golden undertone, which is classified as *warm*. The skin colour can be either creamy ivory, peachy pink, or peach-beige. The skin almost looks clear as glass, and freckles are a natural attribute. The ivory springs appears to have golden flecks or highlights to the skin, while the peachy spring is likely to have peachy-pink cheeks. Some springs are very pinkish and can be confused with summers. Look at the parts of your body that do not blush to see whether you are peach or truly pink.

The eye colour of spring women can be blue with white rays, aqua, bright blue with a turquoise tone, clear blue with possible brown flecks, clear green with possible golden flecks, light golden brown.

Hair colours of the spring colour personality can be golden blonde, strawberry, bright red, or golden brown. Some even have vivid carrot-red hair. Many springs are blonde in childhood, ranging from golden to honey to strawberry, but their hair often darkens with age. Some have very dark brown hair. Ash-tone hair is not spring. Grey does not arrive gracefully on springs, and she will be wise to keep her hair dyed to keep the youthful colour.

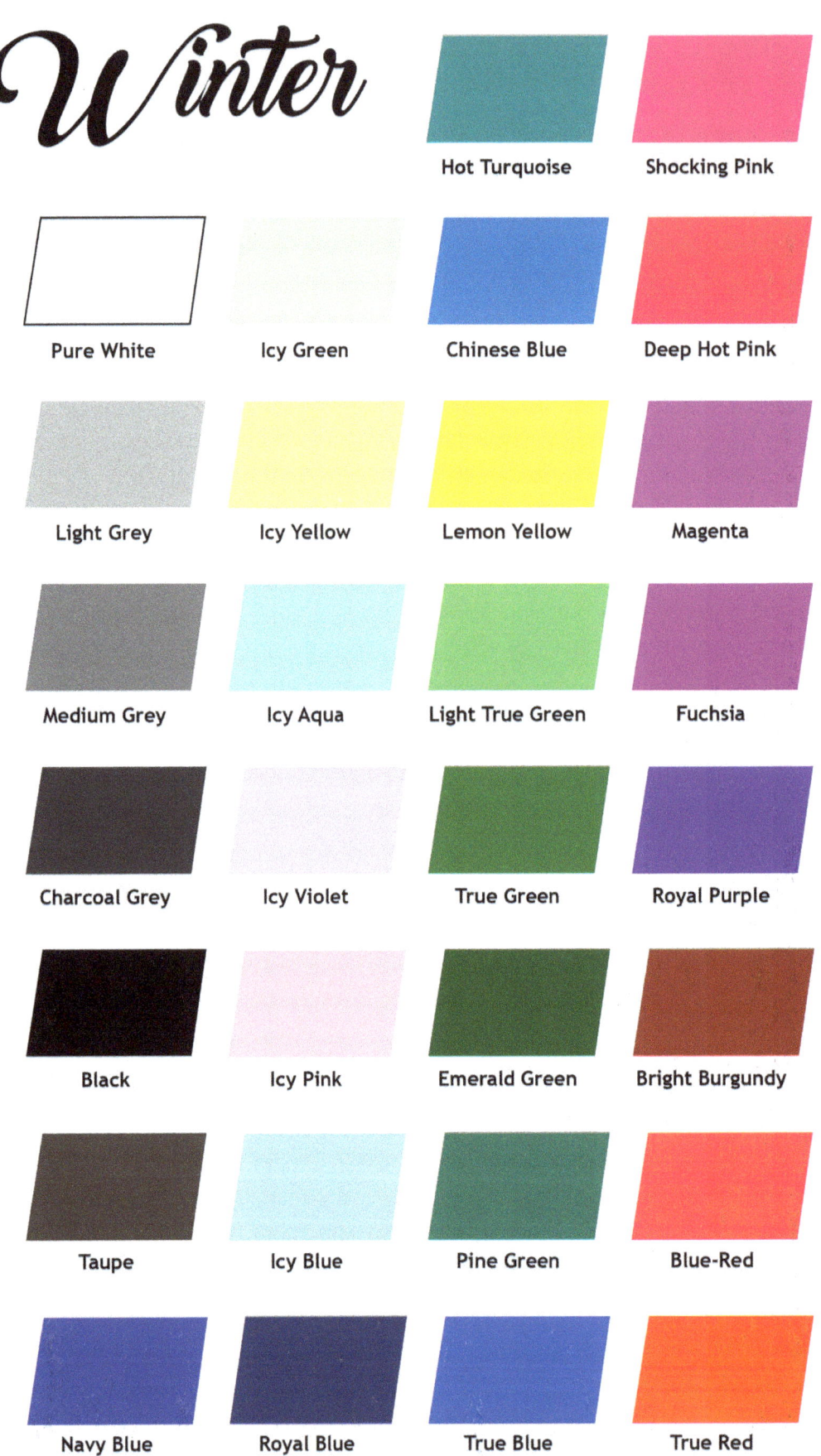

Winter colour palette.

Summer

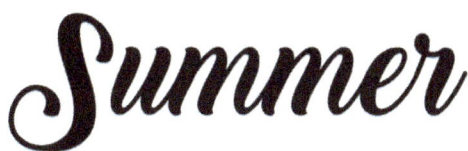

Light Lemon Yellow

Lavender

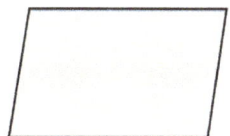
Soft White

Powder Blue

Powder Pink

Orchid

Rose-Beige

Sky Blue

Pastel Pink

Mauve

Cocoa

Medium Blue

Rose Pink

Raspberry

Rose-Brown

Periwinkle Blue

Deep Rose

Soft Fuchsia

Light Blue-Grey

Pastel Aqua

Watermelon

Plum

Charcoal Blue-Grey

Pastel Blue-Green

Blue-Red

Burgundy

Grey Navy

Grey-Blue

Medium Blue-Green

Deep Blue-Green

Summer colour palette.

Autumn

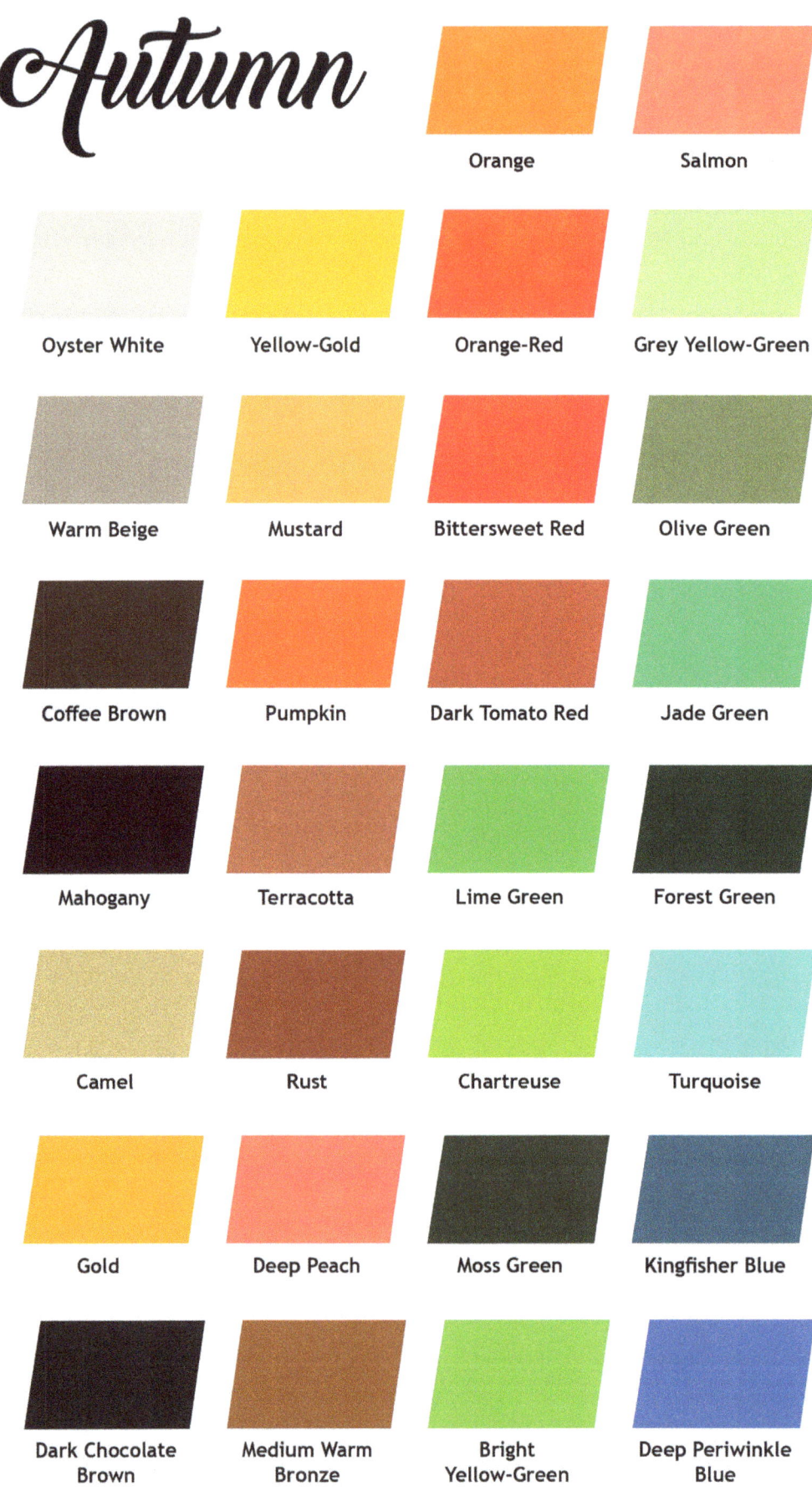

Autumn colour palette.

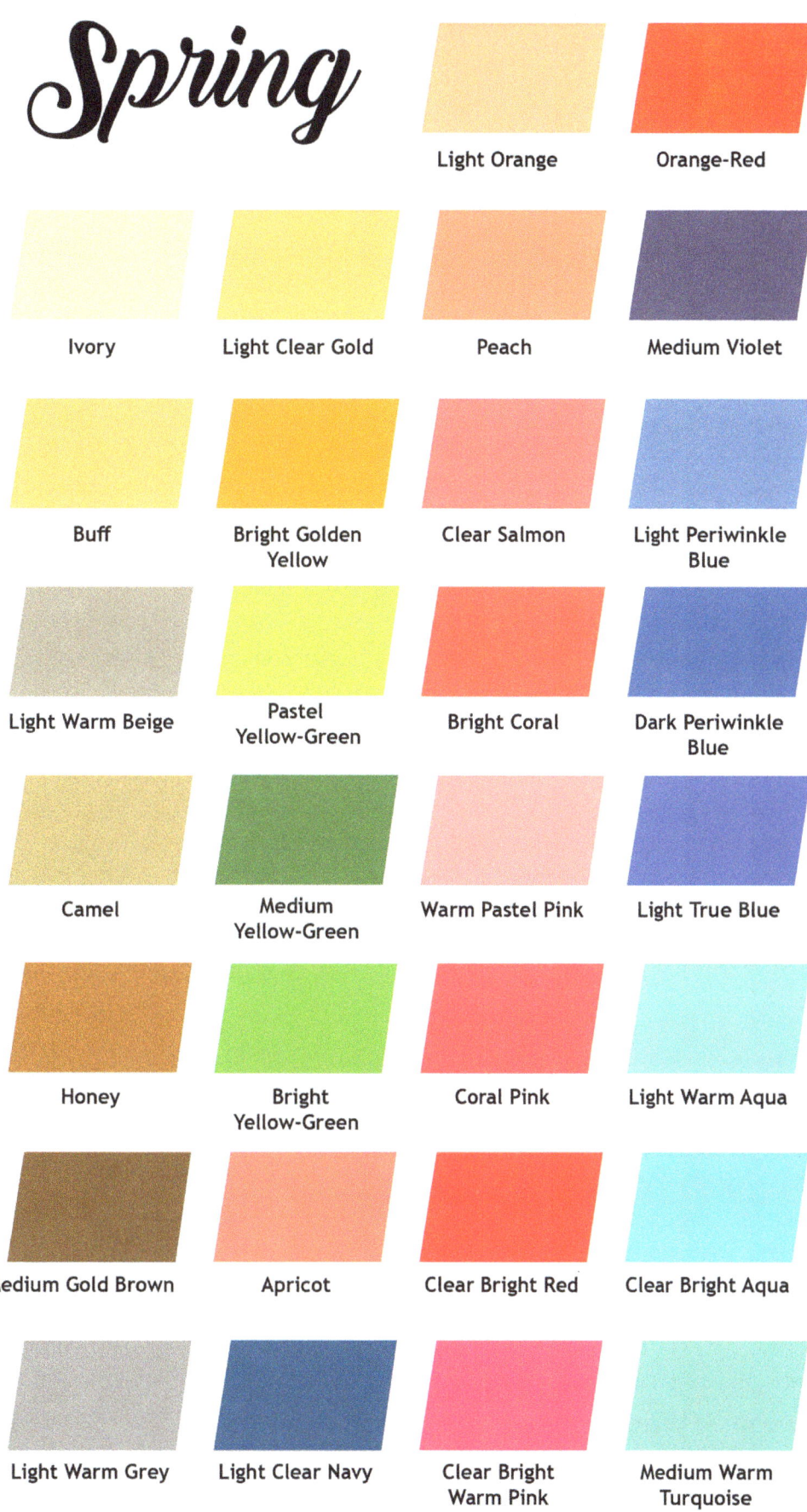

Spring colour palette.

Flow Colour Analysis

The flow colour analysis consists of twelve colour seasons and is based on the original four colour season theory from the *Color Me Beautiful* system by Carole Jackson. Although it was a breakthrough, it only takes into account your lightness or depth and warmth or coolness. Since then it has been discovered that there is more to your colouring than just those characteristics. Our main colour season never changes with age. The colours tend to become more soft and cool, less vivid and intense, but if you maintain your hair colour by covering greys, the effect will not be so evident.

The problem is that some women do not fit neatly into one of the four seasons, and the flow colour analysis recognizes that a person may have colouring characteristics from more than one season. A woman still has one primary season, but also has elements of another season, and the flow colour analysis takes this into account. For example, a woman who has brown to black hair, dark-brown eyes, and an olive skin will be mainly a winter according to the four main seasons, but will flow towards autumn. She will then be a deep winter. The deep winter's colours include all the main winter colours and some of the autumn range, such as olive and khaki, to complement her skin.

The solution to the problem is Munsell's three-dimensional colour theory. Munsell's colour model demonstrates relationships between full-spectrum hues (colour families) as well as tints (value) and shades (chroma).

Chroma distinguishes strong, saturated colours from weak greyish ones.

- high chroma: rich and clear
- low chroma: dull or muted

Adding 'chroma' to the four colour season theory created a more accurate twelve colour season theory, called the flow colour analysis.

Understanding a few characteristics of colour will help you make more informed colour choices when you buy clothes. When we see colours of an object, we think it is red or blue, bright or dark, and vivid or dull. The sensation that we feel when we think an object is 'red or blue' is distinguished in terms of hue. 'Bright or dark' is understood as colour value (lightness), and 'vivid or dull' is identified as chroma or saturation. These three elements are called the three attributes of colour and were created by Professor Albert Munsell.

Hue

Hue is the name of the colour, the attribute of a colour by which it is discernible as red, green, blue, yellow, etc. Each colour is either warm or cool.

Colour Value

Designates the brightness of a colour. Colours vary from dark to light. A colour can be described as light, medium-light, medium, medium–dark, and dark.

Chroma or Saturation

The intensity of a colour is chroma. When colour is fully saturated, the colour is considered in its purest or truest version. The primary colours red, blue, and yellow are considered the truest versions as they are fully saturated. As the saturation increases, the colours appear to be more pure. As the saturation decreases, the colours appear to be more washed-out or pale. Brightness of the colour is controlled by the amount of white mixed in the hue.

How These Values Work in the Twelve Flow Colours

There are six main qualities that you might have in your colouring: Warm, cool, dark (deep), light, clear, muted (soft).

Once you find your dominant characteristic, you will be on your way to find your best colours to wear. Depending on the time of year and your level of tan, you may flow between the seasons of your dominant characteristic.

Determining Your Dominant Characteristics

Look at yourself from shoulders up in a larger mirror with good natural lighting. Leave your hair down unless it is dyed very differently from its natural colour. In this case, you can use a cap to hide your hair colour. Wear no make-up. The features to focus on are your hair (if your natural colour), eyes, and skin tone.

Look for one of the following six features:

1. *Cool*: Blue-based skin colour; no yellow or golden undertones, pink or rosy glow on the cheeks. Eyes are most often blue, but grey is common too.
2. *Warm*: Yellow-based skin colour; no blue undertones. Red hair and green or blue eyes are common. Other warm hair colours are found, too.
3. *Clear*: Bright, clear colours; no single face feature is muted or dusty. Eyes are often clear and sparkly.
4. *Deep*: Strong, rich, dark colouring. Dark hair and eyes. Skin may or may not be dark.
5. *Light*: Very light. Light eyes and hair. They're usually a natural blonde in childhood.
6. *Muted*: Soft, dusty colours; nothing bright and overpowering. There is little contrast between the eyes, skin, and hair.

Determine Your Secondary Characteristic

After you have determined your dominant characteristics, you now have to decide if 'warmer' or 'cooler' colours look best on you. If 'warm' or 'cool' is already your dominant characteristic, decide whether 'clear' or 'muted' colours will look best by looking at the previous six features. After finishing these two steps, you will find your season in the flow seasonal table.

Dominant Characteristics	Secondary Characteristics	Your Season Type
Light + Warm	=	Light Spring
Clear + Warm	=	Clear Spring
Warm + Clear	=	Warm Spring
Light + Cool	=	Light Summer
Muted + Cool	=	Soft Summer
Cool + Muted	=	Cool Summer
Deep + Warm	=	Deep Autumn
Muted + Warm	=	Soft Autumn
Warm + Muted	=	Warm Autumn
Deep + Cool	=	Deep Winter
Clear + Cool	=	Clear Winter
Cool + Clear	=	Cool Winter

Table of flow seasons.
Source: www.colormepretty.co

The Twelve Flow Seasons

1. Light Spring
2. Clear Spring
3. Warm Spring
4. Light Summer
5. Soft Summer
6. Cool Summer
7. Deep Autumn
8. Soft Autumn
9. Warm Autumn
10. Deep Winter
11. Clear Winter
12. Cool Winte

Each woman will have one of the following six dominant characteristics:

- Cool: - winter or summer with cool skin, hair, and eyes.
- Warm: - autumn or spring with warm skin, hair, and eyes.
- Clear: - winter or spring with stunning eyes (many celebrities are clears).
- Deep: - winter or autumn with dark hair and eyes and warm skin.
- Light: - spring and summer with light skin, hair, and eyes.
- Soft muted: - summer or autumn with a velvety or chocolatey look, heavy neutral looks or light and neutral look.

After numerous research efforts, I could not discover who developed the twelve flow seasons. Image consultants around the world are using this system, which gives a more accurate season selection to accommodate most of the people in the first quarter of the twenty-first century. Following are the twelve flow seasons described in more detail.

Light

There are two light seasons, spring and summer.

While spring is warm and bright, summer is cool and muted. The light characteristic means that your colouring appears light, fresh, and delicate with a complete lack of dark features. Light springs will appear more rich and shiny, while light summers have a more soft and neutral look. If you are a light, steer clear of dark and saturated colours in your clothing.

Light Spring

Light spring falls on the border of the spring and the summer seasons. The light spring is the lightest of all the spring seasons. Because your features are so delicate, you have to steer away from wearing dark saturated colours. You can wear the light colours of the spring palette.

Most light springs would have had fair hair colours as children which turned darker over the years to medium golden blonde or brown. Because of your light-golden undertones, your jewellery colours are light gold, rose gold, light bronze, light copper, peach/pink/white stones or diamonds.

- *eyes*: blue, green, light hazel
- *hair*: light to medium golden blonde, light to medium golden brown
- *skin*: pale ivory with a peachy tone, ivory with a peachy tone, tanned ivory with peachy tone

Light Summer

Light summer is a blend between summer and spring. You are light and have a cool undertone. All features are light and cool, such as a cool blue, green, or grey eyes. The overall look of the light summer is soft, delicate, and elegant.

Avoid pure black and saturated colours that will be too strong for your light features. Cool-toned jewellery will blend in well with your soft skin, hair, and eye colour. Because of your cool undertone, your jewellery colours are silver, white gold, diamonds, and light stones.

- *eyes*: blue, green, blue-grey, green-grey
- *hair*: light to medium ash blonde, light ash brown, pale and soft red, grey blonde, cool grey
- *skin*: light ivory, very pale beige, soft beige, cool pink-toned beige, rosy beige

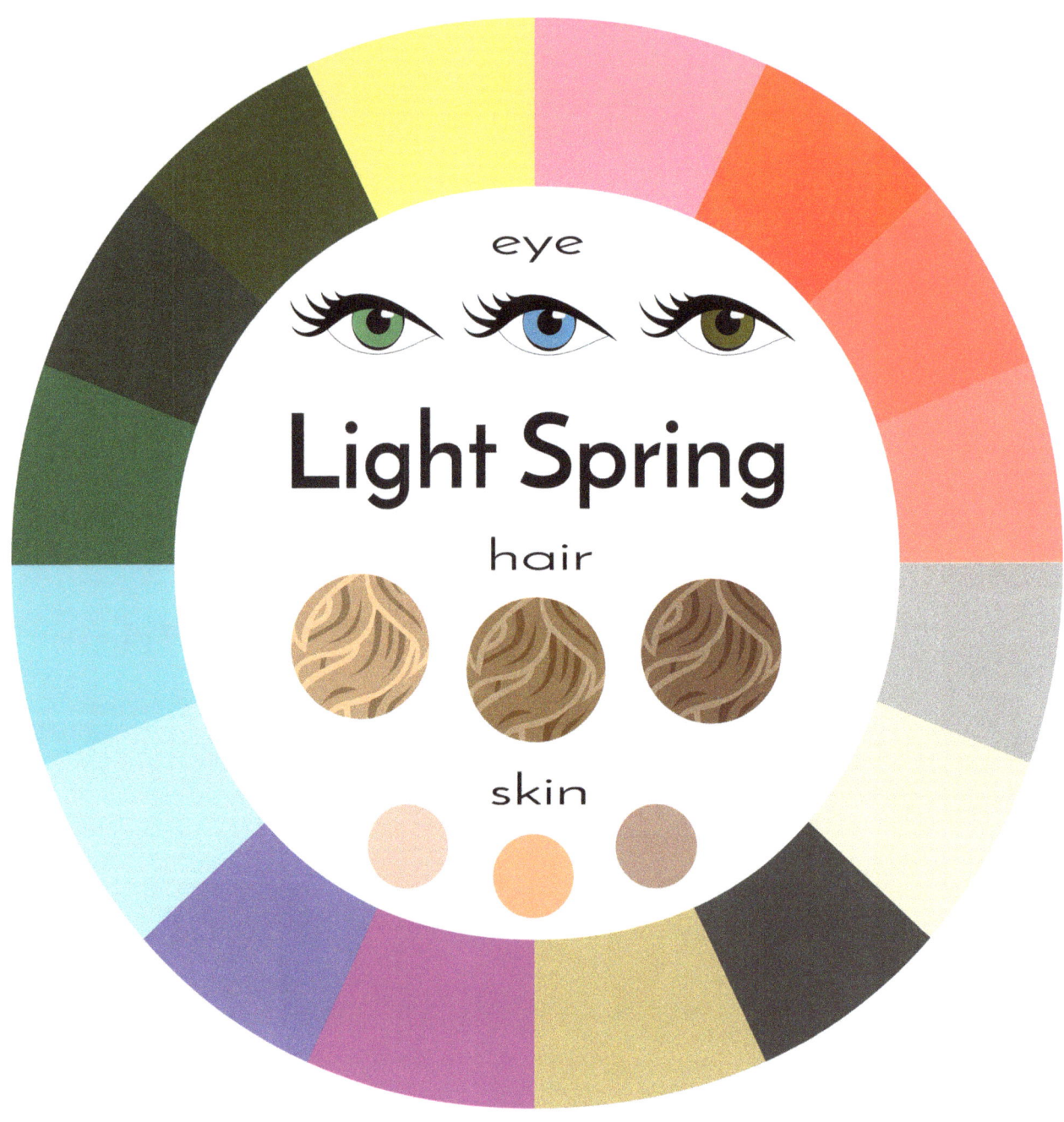

Colours for the Light Spring

Start at twelve o'clock and move in a clockwise direction: light pink, clear red, coral, clear salmon, warm light grey, cream, khaki, camel, fuchsia, light iris purple, powder blue, clear aqua, emerald green, moss green, light warm moss green, light yellow.

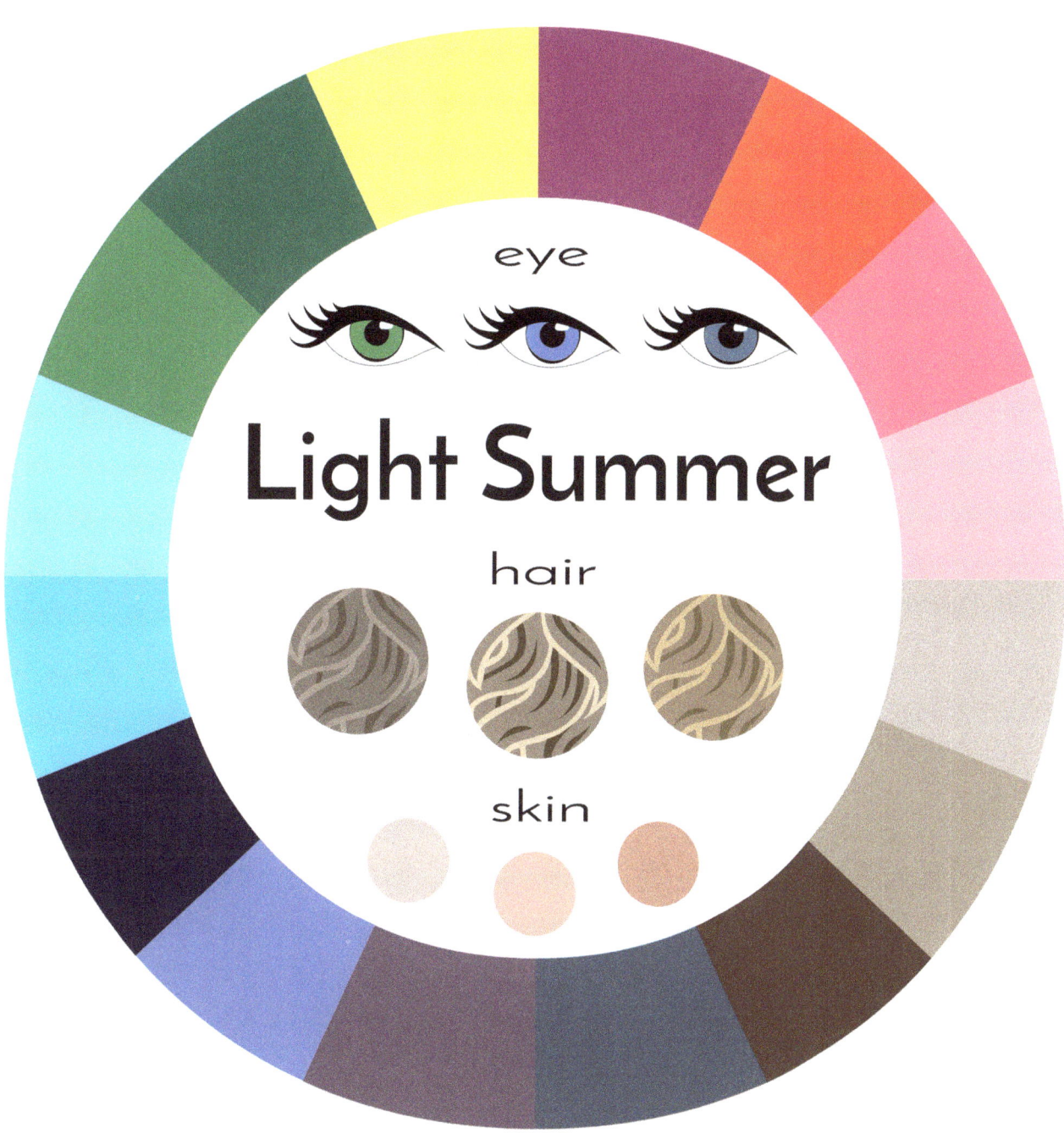

Colours for the Light Summer

Start at twelve o'clock and move in a clockwise direction: red violet, strawberry red, rose pink, shell pink, pale-pink beige, beige khaki, soft cocoa, cool grey, dusty purple, periwinkle, navy, sky blue, light aqua, sea green, spruce, light yellow.

Deep

There are two deep seasons, autumn and winter.

While autumn is warm and soft, winter is cool and bright. People with the deep characteristic have a deep, dark, rich colouring with absolutely no light features except for very pale skin tones.

Your colouring appears rich and bold. Deep winters have more cool, crisp saturation in their colouring and may have very light skin, while deep autumns have more warmth and softness to all their features. If you are a deep autumn, stay away from light and delicate colours in your clothing.

Deep Autumn

Your main season is autumn that flows into winter. You have a golden skin undertone, but not as much contrast the winters have. Because of your golden undertones, your best jewellery choices are gold, bronze and copper, diamond, yellow, or peach stones.

You can wear all the warm colours on the autumn colour palette. As your skin and hair have warm tones, avoid wearing pure black and pure white. Rather, wear a warm off-white or cream and wear black shade under the pure black, such as ebony or raven black.

- *eyes*: dark brown, dark green, dark hazel
- *hair*: dark brown, chestnut, deep chestnut
- *skin*: ivory, golden beige, bronze

Deep Winter

Your dominant features are deep and dark. Most women fall in this category. Because of your deep and dark features, you will look good in primary colours on the colour wheel, pure white, and pure black.

Winters are the only seasons that can wear pure black and white with success, as they enhance their skin tone and bring it to life. Since you have cool features, your best jewellery colours are silver, white gold, diamonds or cool-coloured stones, black, charcoal, and royal blue.

- *eyes*: black, black–brown, dark-hazel
- *hair*: black, black–brown, medium brown, steel grey, salt and pepper
- *skin*: very pale beige, beige, olive, black–brown, black

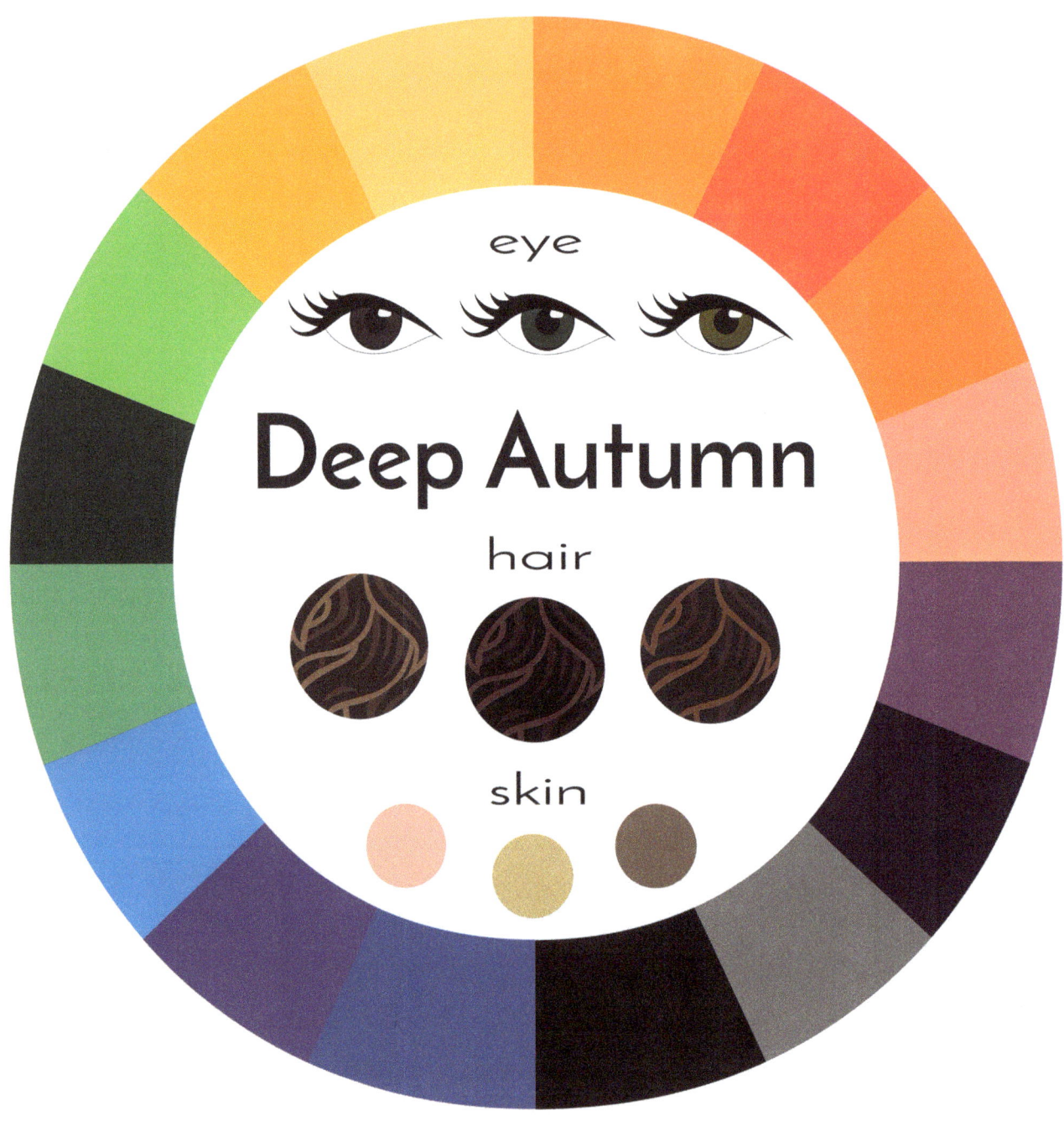

Colours for the Deep Autumn

Start at twelve o'clock and move in a clockwise direction: orange, tomato red, tangerine, light salmon, light plum, dark plum, medium taupe, black, clear navy, deep violet, china blue, emerald green, dark green, lime green, amber, light golden yellow.

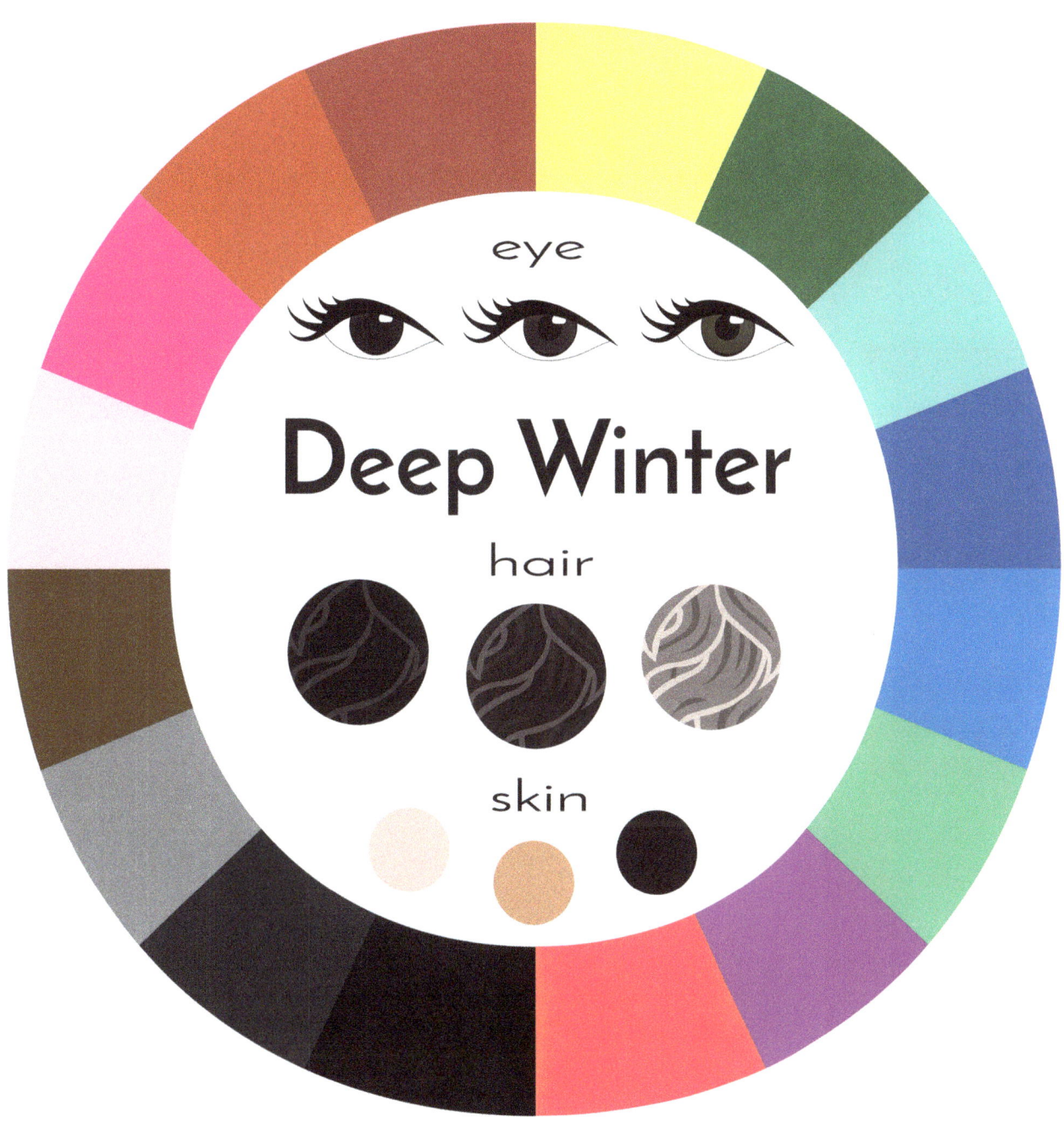

Colours for the Deep Winter

Start at twelve o'clock and move in a clockwise direction: light yellow, forest green, turquoise, bright navy, bright blue, mint, warm purple, blue–red, black, charcoal, medium grey, sepia, icy pink, hot pink, true cool red, carnelian.

Clear

There are two clear seasons, spring and winter.

While spring is warm and light, winter is cool and deep. Those with clear colouring tend to have a striking, vivid look. Skin has a translucent quality to it, and eyes are clear, sparkly, and bright. Their overall look has a lot of saturation and contrast. For those with the clear characteristic, the first thing you will usually notice about them is their eyes. If you are a clear, wearing darks and lights together will emphasize your high contrast even more.

Clear Spring

The clear spring is a blend of spring and winter. Many clears had blonde hair as a child and continued their blonde hair as an adult. Other clears' hair change to a medium brown or brown-black during their late teens, or early twenties. Your overwhelming tone is warm; therefore, your best jewellery colours are gold, bronze, copper, diamond, and warm -toned stones.

Keep the colours that you wear clear and bright. Avoid dark, dusty, and pale colours, which will make you look dull. Clear spring is the only spring on the twelve flow seasons that can wear black successfully, but stick with a black shade that is warmer than a true/dark black.

- *eyes*: green, turquoise blue, topaz
- *hair*: medium golden brown, dark golden brown, brown-black (possibly with red
- highlights)
- *skin*: porcelain, light ivory, peach, bronze, warm deep brown, brown-black

Clear Winter

Your main season is a winter that flows into spring. The clear winter's features are clear and bright with high contrast between the eyes, skin tone, and hair colour. Wear colours that are clear with contrasting qualities. Because you are a winter with a cool undertone, you can wear true black and white successfully.

Avoid warm shades and muted colours, such as orange, corals, mustard, and warm browns. Your best jewellery colours are silver, white gold, rose gold, diamonds, blue sapphire, red ruby, emerald green, even pink stones.

- *eyes*: emerald green, bright blue, violet
- *hair*: medium brown, dark brown, black with blue or ash tints
- *skin*: milky-white to light and neutral beige, pale olive, deep brown, black

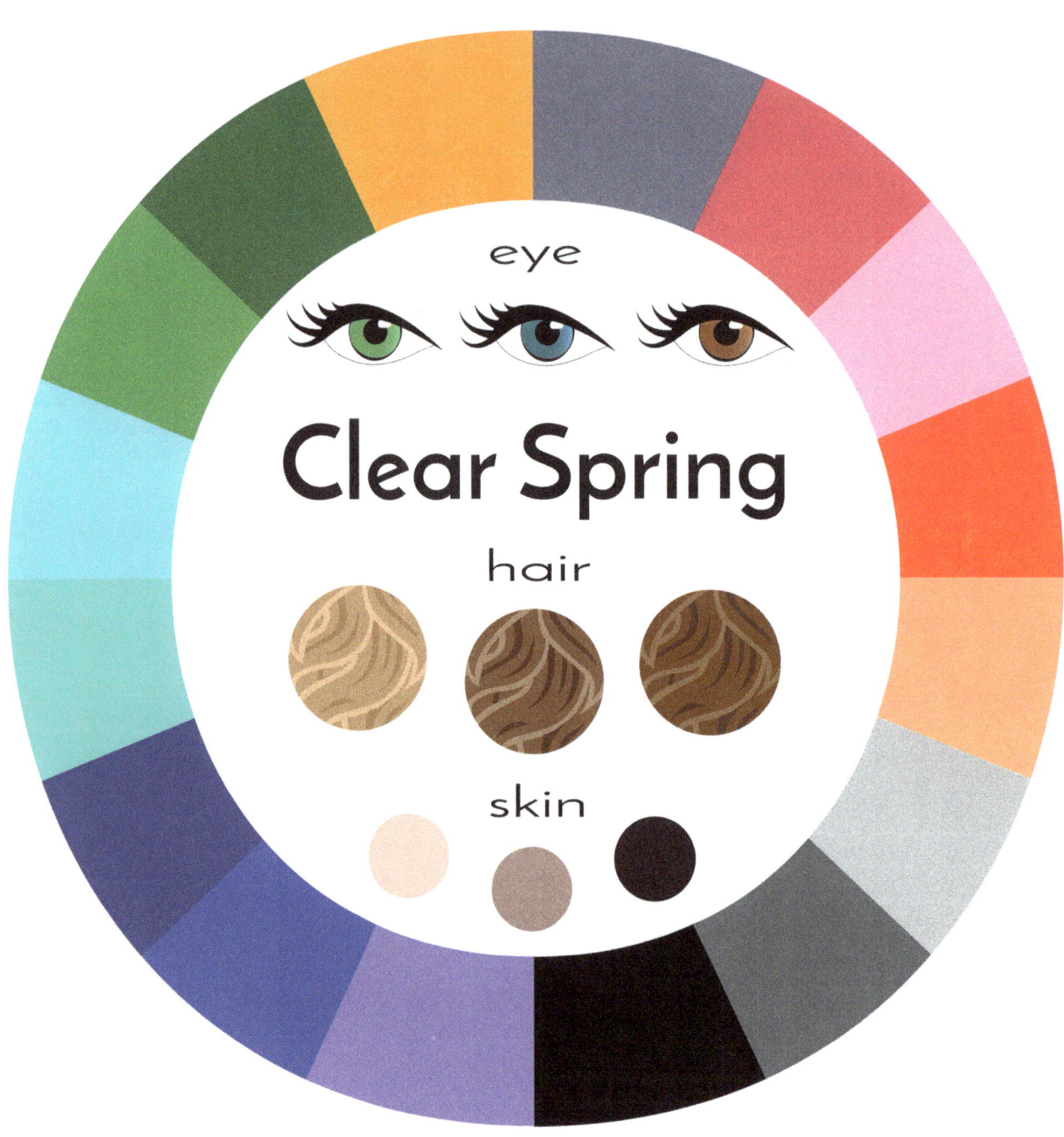

Colours for the Clear Spring

Start at twelve o'clock and move in a clockwise direction: purple grey, dark rose pink, pastel pink, red-orange, peach, light grey, light charcoal, black, light iris purple, true blue, clear navy, robin egg blue, aqua, green, dark green, marigold.

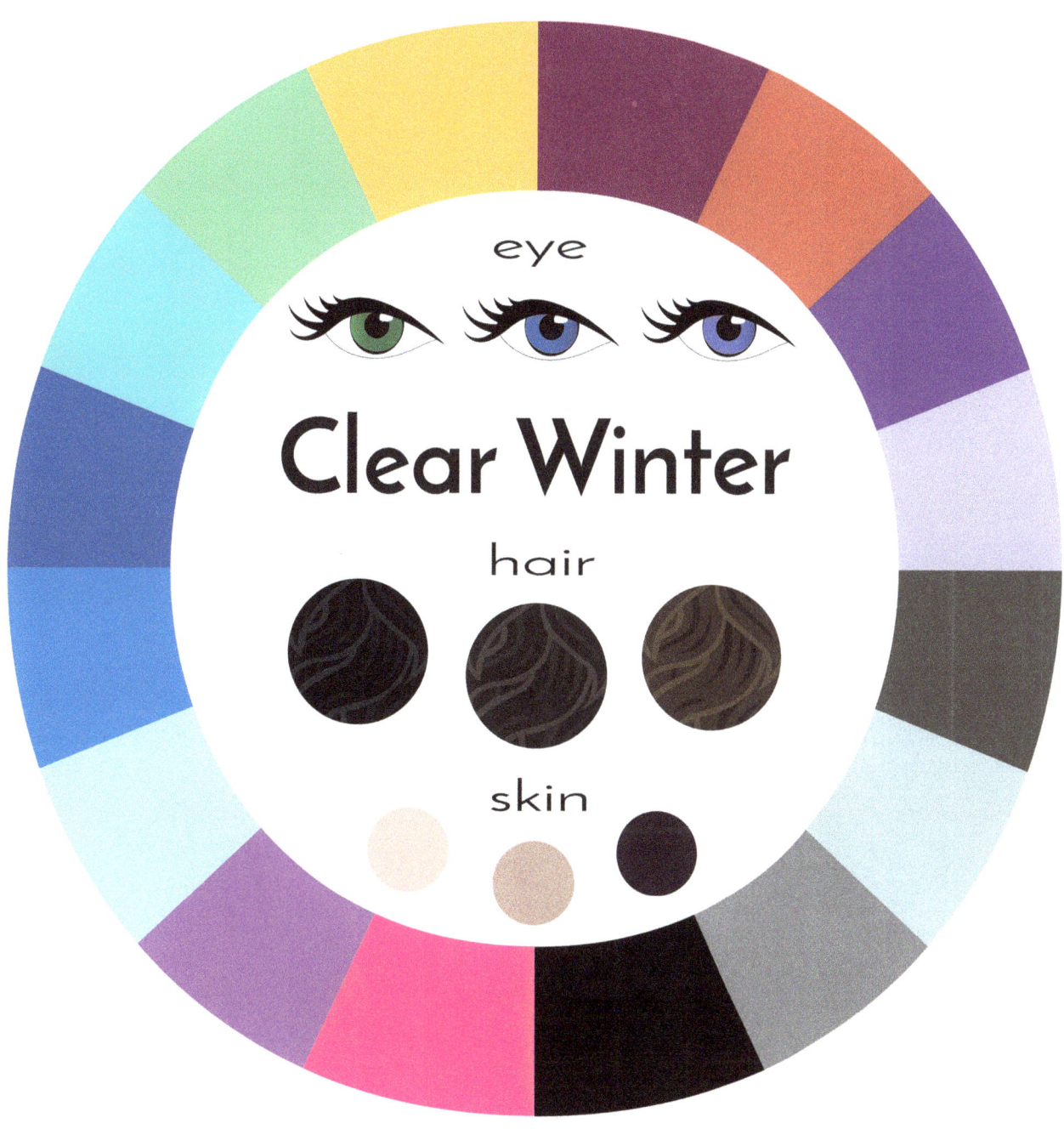

Colours for the Clear Winter

Start at twelve o'clock and move in a clockwise direction: dark raspberry, dark–salmon, dark violet, icy lavender, taupe, icy grey, medium grey, black, hot pink, orchid, icy blue, bright blue, bright navy, aqua, light emerald green, light-golden yellow.

Soft

There are two soft seasons, summer and autumn.

While summer is light and cool, autumn is deep and warm. If you have soft colouring, you tend to have a low level of saturation and contrast between your hair, eyes, and skin, and you may appear somewhat neutral.

Your overall look is serene and down-to-earth. If you are a soft, keep your clothing colours within a few levels or shades of each other, that will make you glow.

Soft Summer

The soft summer is a blend of summer and autumn. Summers are always soft/muted, light, and cool. Therefore, your colours should be light with more of a cool tone. Your features do not have a huge contrast between them and are usually colours that blend in with one another.

As a soft summer, you are limited to the soft, muted colours of the summer palette. Because of your cool undertone, your best jewellery colours are silver, white gold, diamonds, and light stones.

- *eyes*: blue-grey, green–hazel, brown-hazel
- *hair*: light to medium ash-brown colours with possible ash blonde highlights
- *skin*: very pale beige to light neutral beige, pink-toned to rosy beige, medium neutral beige

Soft Autumn

The soft autumn flows into summer. And since the summer season is cool, the soft summer can look quite neutral. If you are an autumn, you are always soft/muted and warm. Again there is not a huge contrast between your features.

You do not have to be limited to colours and can really enjoy any colour of the spectrum, as long as it is soft/muted and with a warm undertone. Because you have more autumn qualities with warm undertone, your best colour jewellery are gold, light bronze, light copper, diamonds, yellow or peachy stones.

- *eyes*: green, blue, grey–green, light brown to light hazel
- *hair*: dark golden blonde to medium brown, brown to medium brown, possibly with blonde or red highlights
- *skin*: ivory, light neutral to neutral beige, medium neutral beige

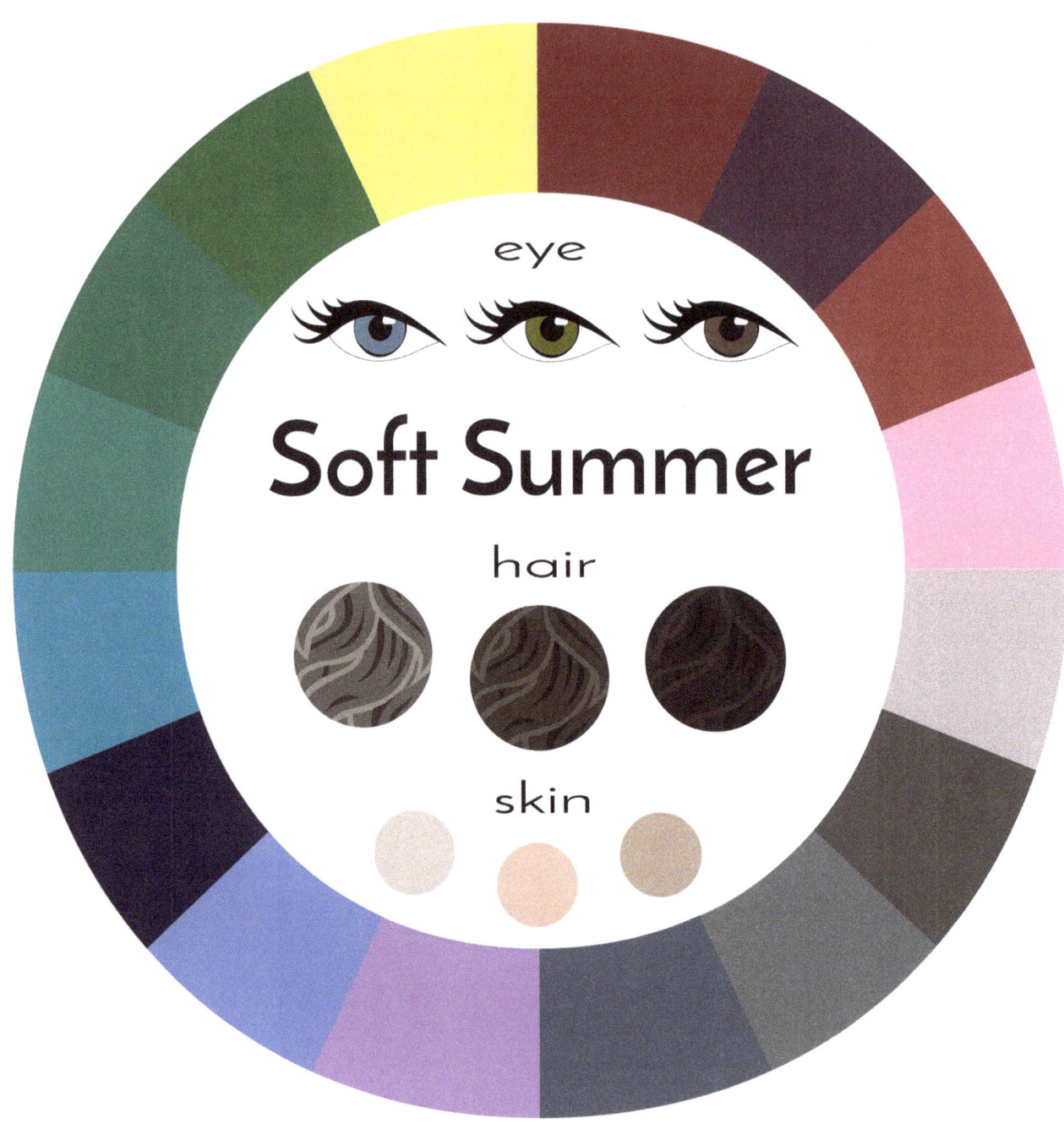

Colours for the Soft Summer

Start at twelve o'clock and move in a clockwise direction: burgundy, deep mauve, deep rose, baby pink, pale-pink beige, taupe, grey, cool grey, lavender, periwinkle, navy, blue teal, pine green, spruce, emerald green, light yellow.

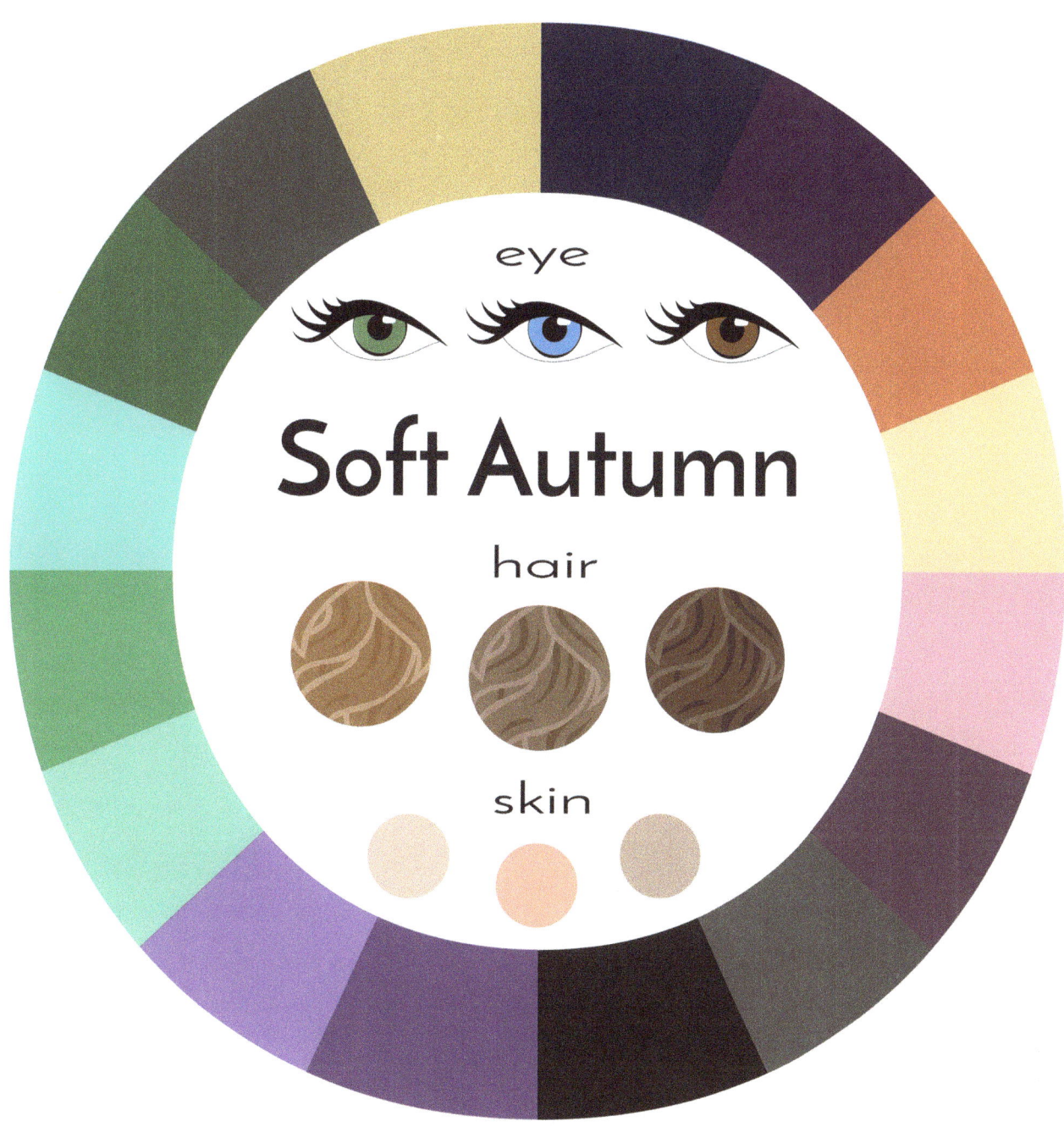

Colours for the Soft Autumn

Start at twelve o'clock and move in a clockwise direction: navy, aubergine, terracotta, buttermilk, dusty pink, warm mauve, taupe, dark chocolate brown, dark amethyst, amethyst, green aqua, emerald, turquoise, light evergreen, khaki, camel.

Warm

There are two warm seasons, spring and autumn.

While spring is light and bright, autumn is deep and muted. As a warm, your colouring gives you an earthy glow; therefore, warm and earthy colours will suit you well.

Keep your clothing colours within a few levels or shades of each other, that will make you glow. Avoid dark, saturated, and cool colours, which will be too much in contrast to your warm features.

Warm Spring

The warm spring flow a bit in the autumn season; therefore, the dominant colour is warm, golden, and clear. You should wear warm colours that are clear and not muted or too bright.

Steer clear from dark, saturated colours like, black and white; they will make you look washed out. Because of your overwhelming warm features, your jewellery colour needs to have warm colours: gold, rose gold, light bronze, light copper, diamond (diamond takes on any colour), emerald, and warm-coloured stones.

- *eyes*: blue, olive green, topaz, light hazel
- *hair*: deep-golden blonde to light golden brown, strawberry blonde, or coppery red
- *skin*: porcelain, ivory, golden beige, bronze

Warm Autumn

When you have obvious cool undertones, then you are definitely not a warm autumn. Red-haired women need to look at the intensity of the red. Redheads with softer features that is more of a cool tone, may be a lighter season.

The autumn colours can be dull on many women but will bring the warm autumns to life. Autumns may find it difficult to determine their exact season. The easiest way to find your perfect colours is when you put it on and it brings out your stunning features. When you look dull or tired, it is definitely not your colours. Your jewellery colours are warm: gold, rose gold, bronze, copper, diamond (diamond takes on any colour), emerald, and warm-coloured stones.

- *eyes*: brown, olive green, dark hazel
- *hair*: deep-golden blonde to medium-golden brown, red or auburn
- *skin*: ivory, golden beige to warm beige, bronze

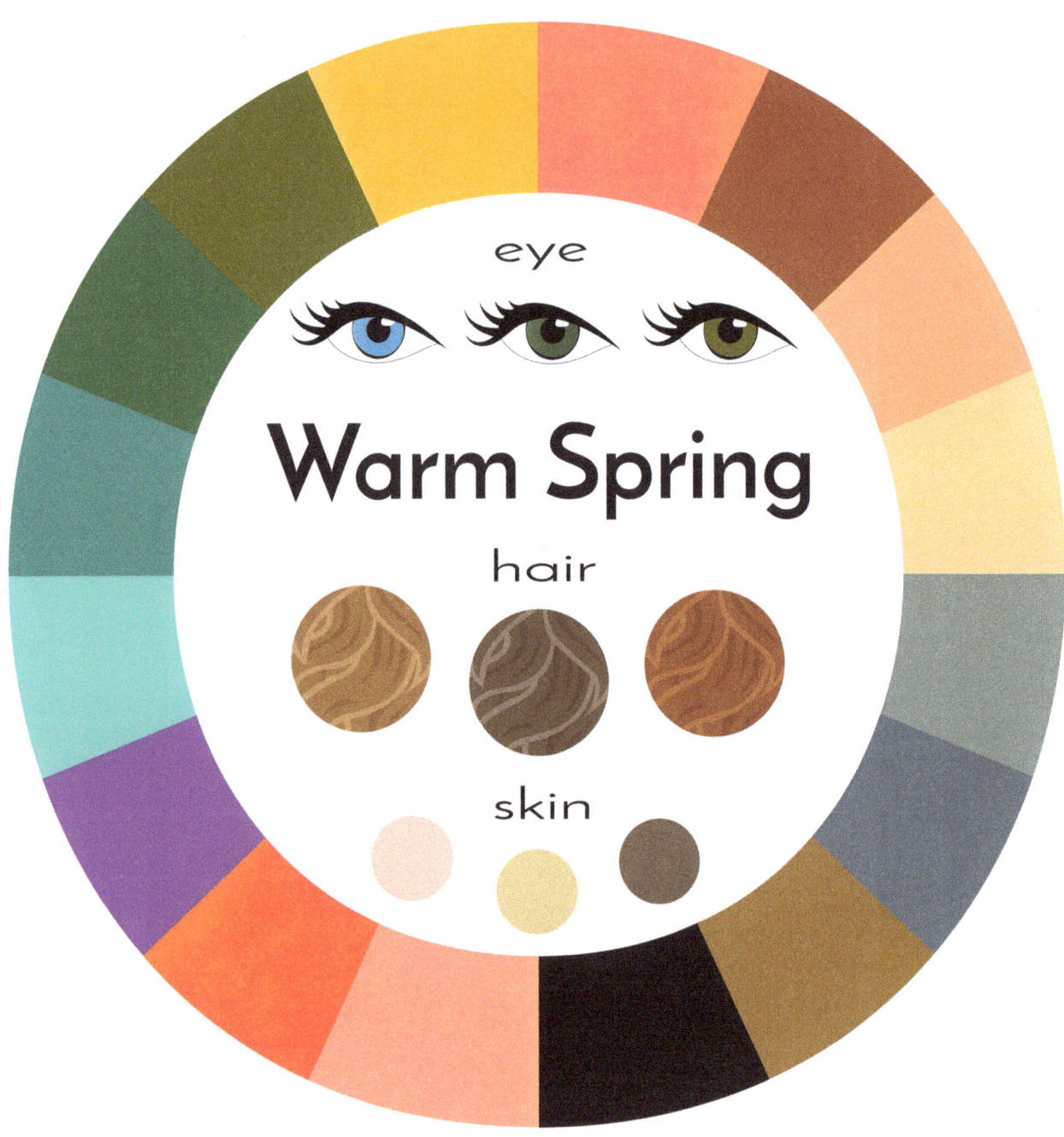

Colours for the Warm Spring

Start at twelve o'clock and move in a clockwise direction: coral, rust, peach, light orange, light grey–green, stone, golden brown, dark brown, light salmon, tomato red, purple, robin egg blue, teal, emerald green, olive, gold yellow.

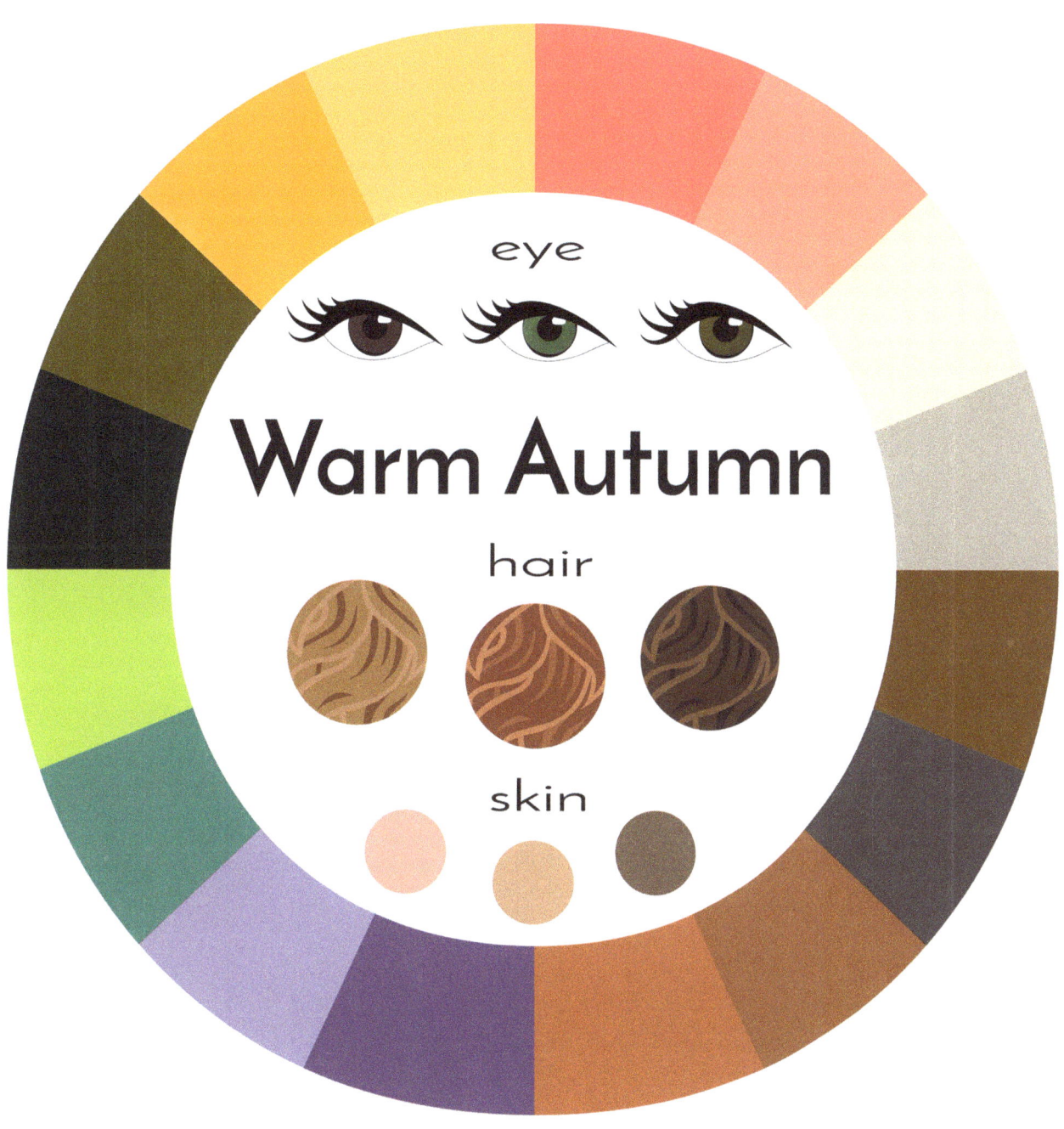

Colours for the Warm Autumn

Start at twelve o'clock and move in a clockwise direction: coral, light salmon, cream, beige, medium brown, brown taupe, sienna, burnt orange, dark amethyst, light amethyst, pine green, light emerald green, dark forest green, olive-moss, amber, light golden yellow.

Cool

There are two cool seasons, summer and winter.

While summer is light and muted, winter is deep and bright. As a cool, you will have greyish, ashy undertones to your features, and you may have a calm and regal appearance.

The cool seasons have bold and dark features; therefore, colours that are cool and vibrant will bring them to life.

Cool Summer

Cool summer flows into the cool winter season. Summer's dominantly colouring is cool, with little to zero warmth to the skin tone. To complement your features, avoid wearing warm and golden colours. Cool colours will accentuate your beautiful cool characteristics. All cool shades of blue will suit you well, even black and white. There are colours that you can wear that overlaps in the cool winter's palette.

Because of your mostly cool features, your jewellery colours are silver, white gold, charcoal, diamond, sapphire, emerald, black, cool and bright pink, and cool red stones.

- *eyes*: blue, grey, charcoal
- *hair*: medium to deep ash-browns with little to no red tones
- *skin*: light to medium neutral beige, cool beige, grey beige, blue-black

Cool Winter

Cool winter does not flow into any warm season but can overlap the cool summer season. Your features are all cool with high contrast; therefore, bold and strong colours will suit you well. Pastel colours may be too soft for you, as they will look too dull on you. Also avoid warm golden colours, such as golden browns and oranges, which also may make you look tired.

Cool winters may have been deep winters when they were younger, because as we age, our features tend to soften and become lighter. As cool winters have no warmth in their features, only cool-coloured jewellery will suit them best, such as silver, white gold, charcoal, black, sapphires, white, diamonds, or any cool-coloured stones.

- *eyes*: blue, violet, charcoal grey
- *hair*: blue-black, silver, salt and pepper (with no red or gold tones)
- *skin*: very pale neutral beige, very pale beige, pale neutral beige, rosy-beige

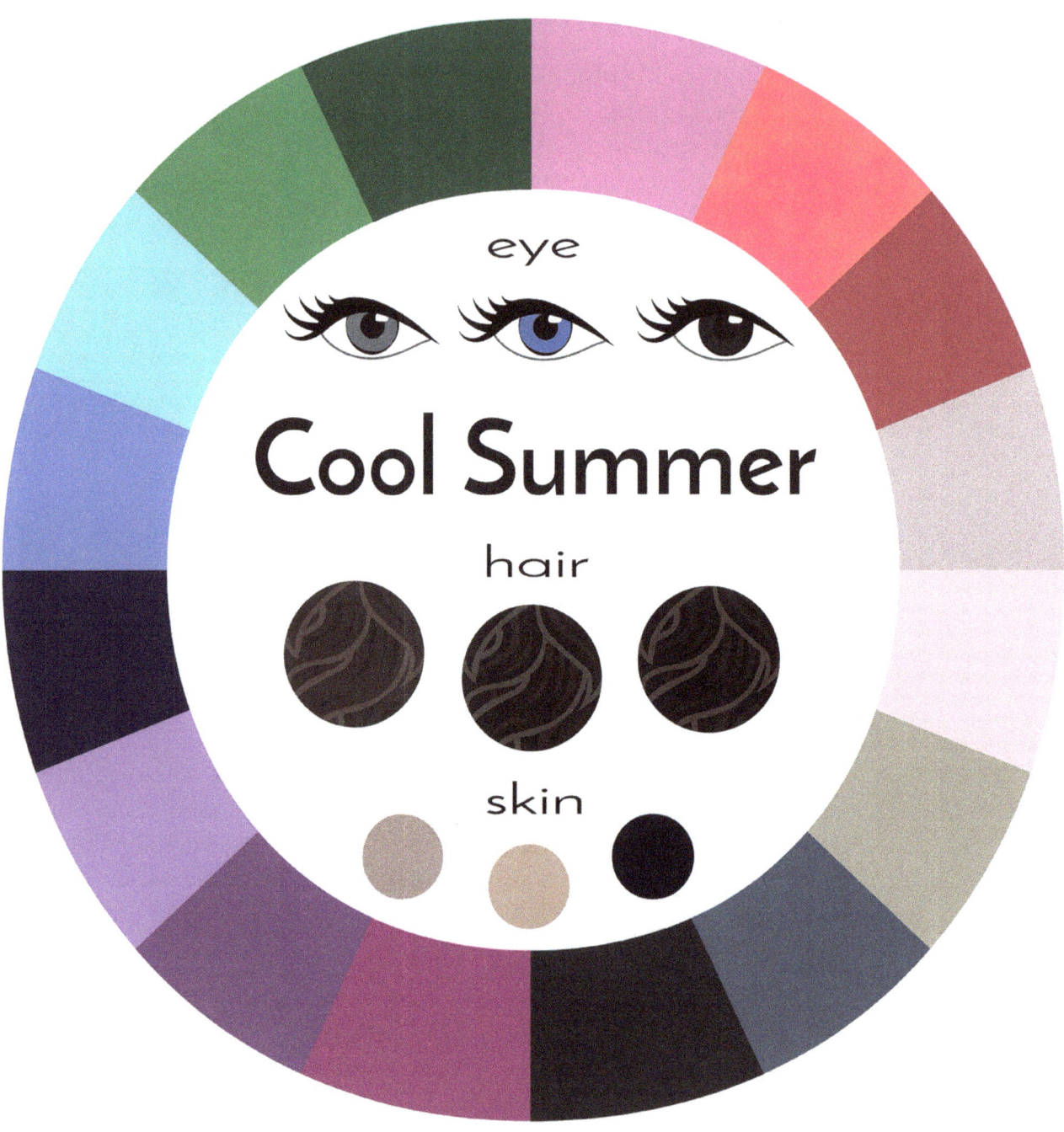

Colours for the Cool Summer

Start at twelve o'clock and move in a clockwise direction: soft fuchsia, rose, raspberry, pale-pink beige, icy pink, cool khaki, cool grey, charcoal, red–violet, hot dusty purple, lavender, navy, periwinkle, light aqua, sea green, evergreen.

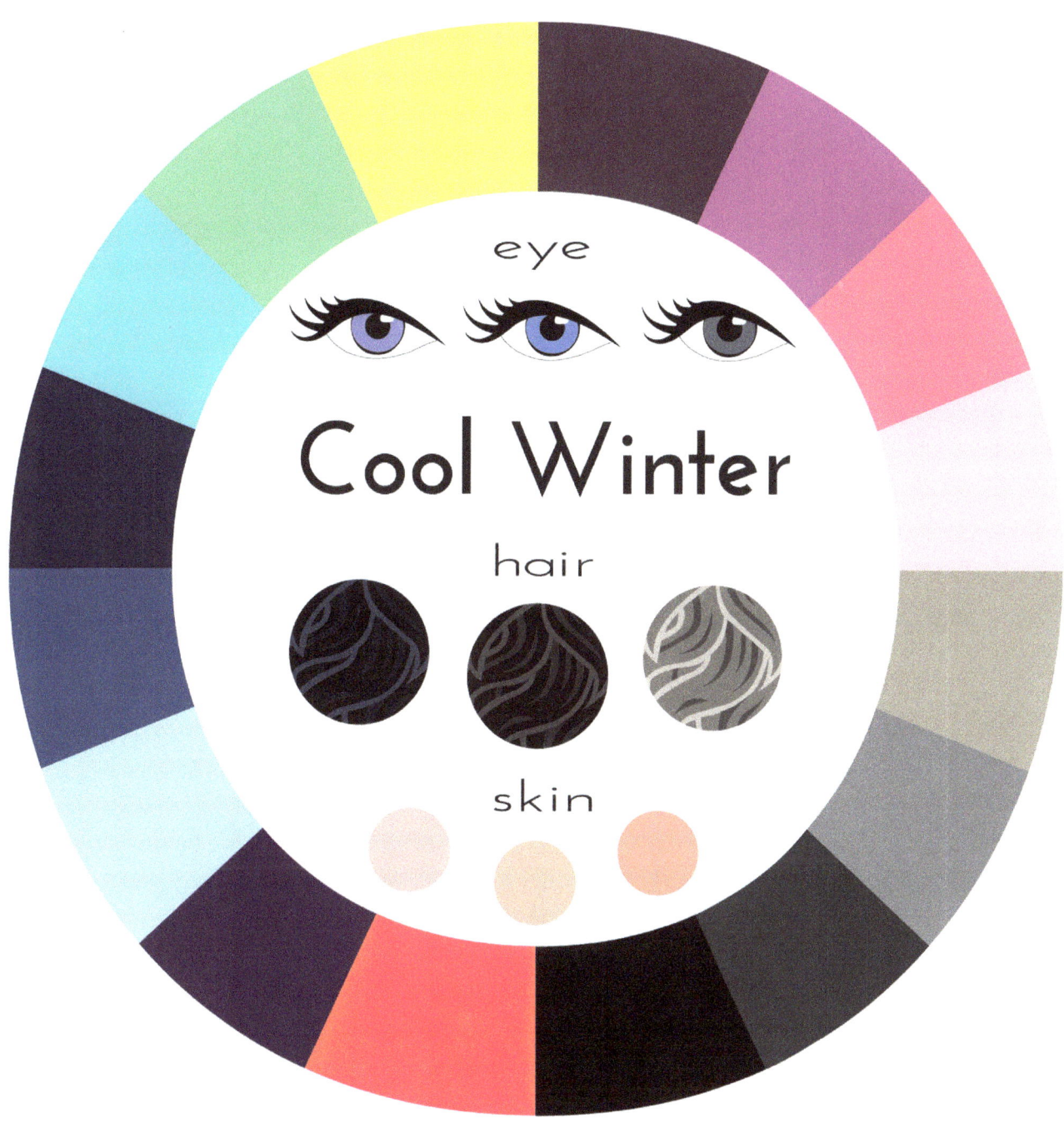

Colours for the Cool Winter

Start at twelve o'clock and move in a clockwise direction: deep mauve, magenta, rose pink, icy pink, cool khaki, medium grey, dark grey, black, blue–red, dark purple, icy blue, royal blue, navy, aqua, light emerald, light yellow.

Get to Know the Colour Wheel

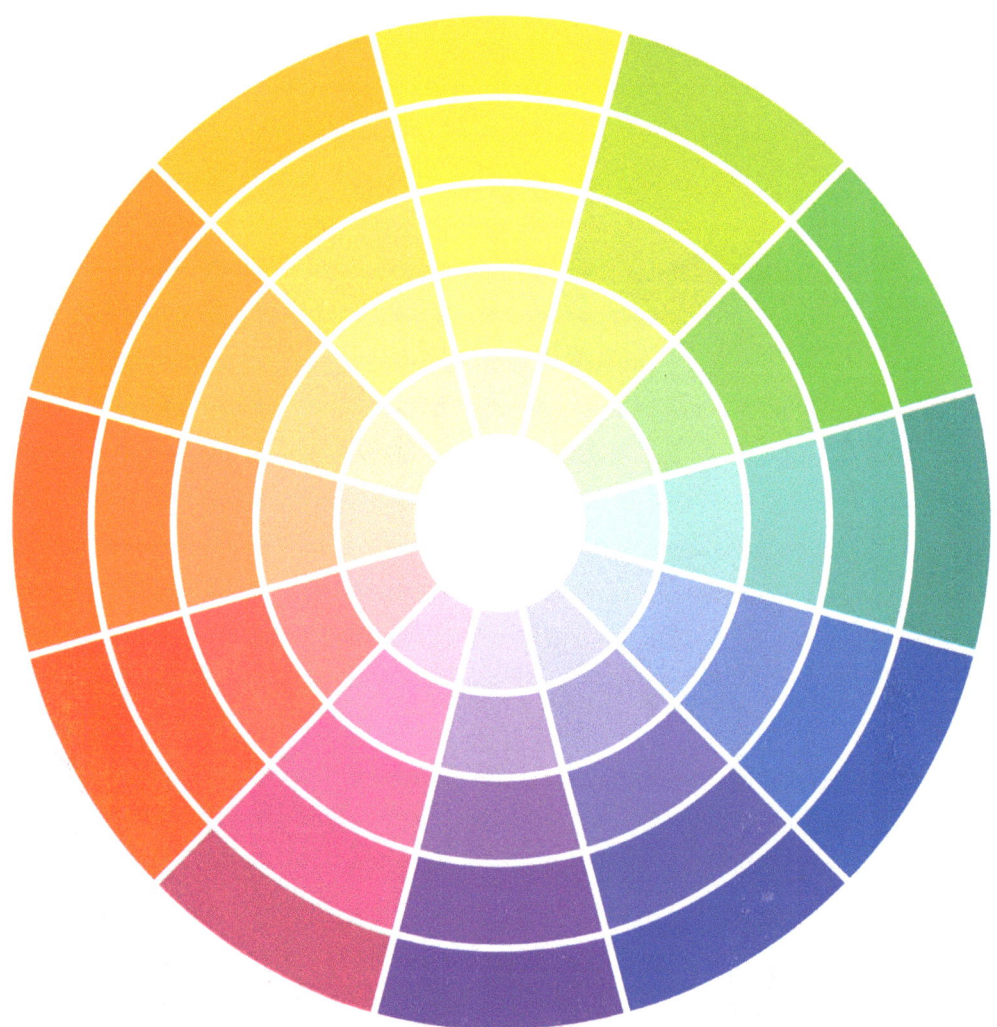

Pick any colour on the colour wheel. Trace your finger over the line to the colour directly opposite, and you have two complementary colours, one warm and one cool. If they complement on the wheel, they will look complementary in your wardrobe. For your most flattering look, place the colour that works best for your skin tone closest to your face and work the other colour in further away. For example, if you have a cool skin tone, choose cool-toned earrings, necklace, and a shirt that will complement your skin tone and features. Wear any warm tones for your skirt, trousers, shoes, or handbag, that is away from your face.

Pick another colour on the wheel. Look to the colour directly to the left and to the right of it. These are the original colour's analogous friends. If they're analogous on the colour wheel, they will work in your outfit. You can now stick to your side of the colour wheel, whether you have a cool or warm undertone, to ensure the best possible palette for your skin. Get to know each, and you'll be less afraid to go for neon colours the next time you buy clothes.

Prescription- and Sunglasses Frames for Each Face Shape

Choose the Best Frame for Your Face Shape

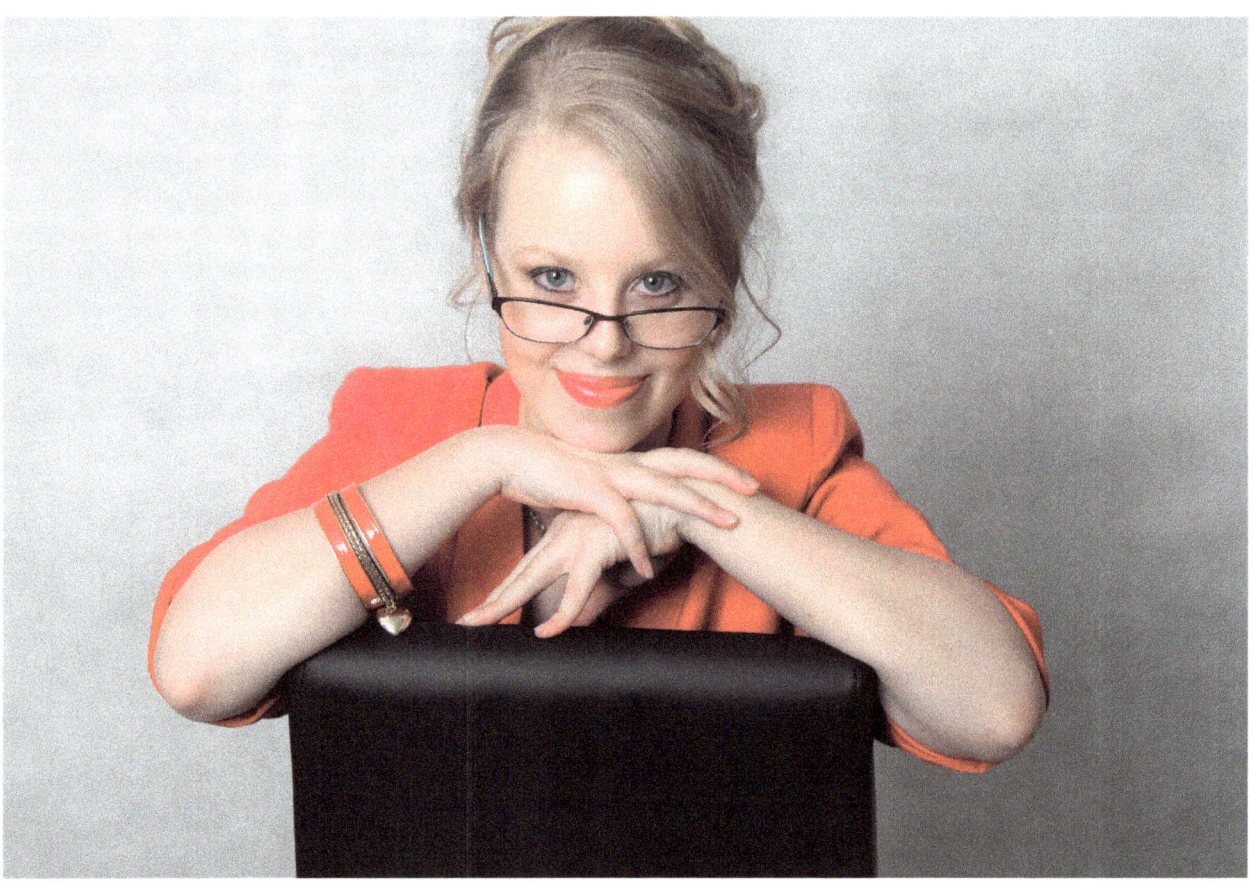

Prescription glasses became quite stylish and women started to use it as fashion accessories, especially amongst fans of high-end designers. Many women choose frames the same way they choose shoes or handbags by selecting different colours and styles to match their wardrobes. Although I do not recommend to only go for the designer brands (especially if your budget does not allow it), it is important that the shape and colour of your prescription glasses fit with your face shape and features. There are plenty of affordable but still good-quality frames. All accessories combined with your outfit and colours make up your final look. You may be stylishly dressed, but if your prescription glasses do not fit your personal features, it can affect your overall look. Rimless glasses are without obvious frames and can blend in without being in contrast with the rest of your outfit colours.

Technology advances has made modern lenses thinner, lighter, and more attractive than ever before. When selecting frames, make sure you analyse your face shape and colouring so that you find the most flattering look for you. While it's fine to admire what a favourite celebrity might be wearing, be mindful that the same style might not be the right look for you. Facial shapes are influenced by the structure of facial bones, that provides a framework for the facial muscles and form features such as eye sockets, cheekbones, and the jawline.

There are nine basic face shapes. Most women will fall into these nine shapes but can also have a combination of two face shapes. For the characteristics of each face shape, refer to the *The Best Necklines for Each Face Shape and Body Shape* section of this book.

How to analyse your face and determine which face shape it is:

- Remove all hair from your face with hair clips or a head-band.
- Look straight into a mirror, and look at all your features and lines in detail.
- You can even draw the outlines of your face with a marker or lipstick directly on your reflection on the mirror. The drawing will give you an indication of the shape. (Clean the mirror afterwards with alcohol wipes or a dampened cloth and vinegar.)

The same way clothing fashions change dramatically around every second year, prescription glasses frames get a makeover as well. Therefore, it will be difficult to show and discuss all the frames out there. In this section, I would like to give you some guidelines so that no matter what selection of frames gets launched, you'll be able to use the advice to narrow down the frames that will fit your face shape and features best. When you go for an eye test, pick around three to six different frames from the advice given in this book. Make your final decision as you fit each one while looking in the mirror. You can follow the same guidelines when choosing sunglasses.

As mentioned, prescription glasses are for many of us a fashion statement, but there are many women dependent on them to see properly. I would like to encourage all fashion enthusiasts who get a new pair of prescription glasses every year, not to throw the old pair in a drawer and forget about it, rather donate it to those who find it hard to afford prescription glasses.

Three main keys to consider when buying frames for your prescription lenses:

1. The frame must not repeat your face shape but rather contrast it.
2. The colour of the frame must complement the colours of your skin, hair, and eyes. For example, when you have blue eyes, the frame can reflect blue.
3. The frame size should be in scale with your face size. Too-big frames are noticed straight away and will throw off the symmetry of your face.

Let's discuss the face shapes and possible eyeglass frames for each:

Oval Face Shape

The oval face shape is considered the ideal face shape because it is balanced and has flattering lines. Any frame will fit this shape, but keep the balanced look by wearing frames that are as wide as, or a bit wider than the broadest part of the face, which is the highest part of the cheekbones.

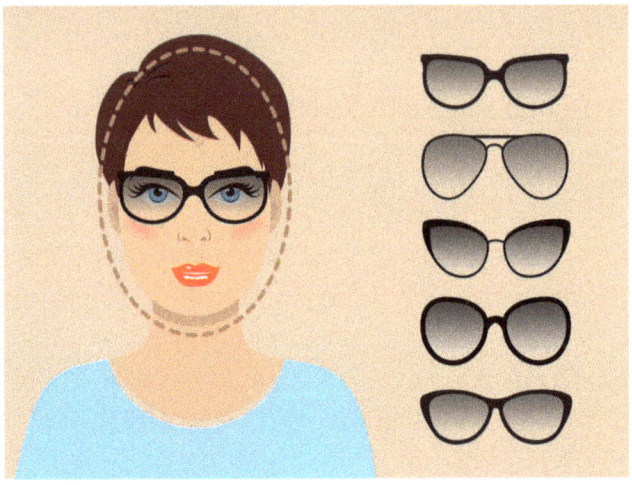

Frames that will suit an oval face have a strong bridge, are wider than the broadest part of the face, and are geometric in shape.

Diamond Face Shape

A diamond face shape has a narrow forehead and a long and narrow jawline that tapers into a point. The cheekbones are broad and the widest part of the face. Highlighting the eyebrow area with distinctive upper rims will give the illusion that the forehead is wider, and it will soften the cheek line.

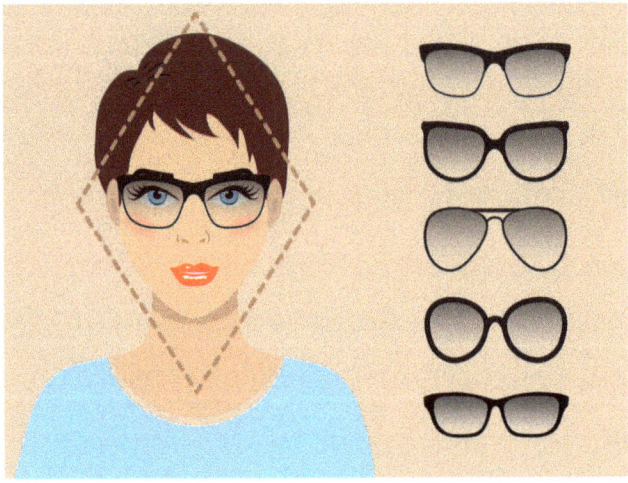

Frames that suit a diamond face have distinctive brow lines, such as cat eye frames and oval frames. Or try rimless frames. Avoid boxy and narrow frames, which will accentuate the width of your cheeks.

Oblong Face Shape

The oblong face is longer than it is wide. To make an oblong face appear shorter and more balanced, wear frames that have more depth than width. Decorative or contrasting temples will make the face appear wider, and a low bridge shortens a long nose. The aim of the frame must be to make the face appear wider.

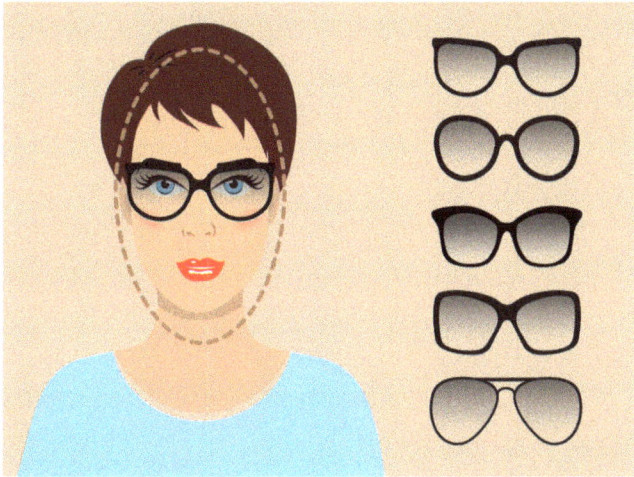

Frames that suit an oblong face are larger squares, round or aviator shapes.

Avoid triangular shapes and short frames, which will accentuate the long, narrow face.

Square Face Shape

The square face shape is equal in length and width. Jawline is strong, broad, and obviously square in appearance. Oval or round frames will balance the face and add a thinner appearance to the strong angles.

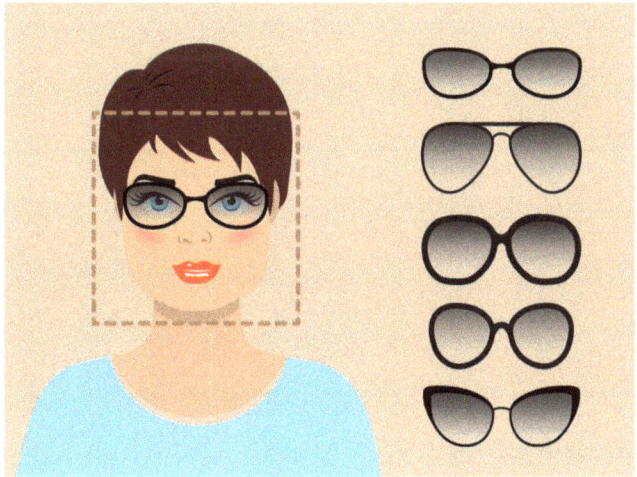

Wear narrow frame styles that have more width than depth and narrow ovals. Cat eye and aviator frames will work as well.

Avoid angular and boxy frames, which will draw attention to the square facial corners.

Heart Face Shape

The face is longer than it is wide. Forehead is wide and round at the hairline. Chin is noticeably pointed, typical like a heart form. Frames with low-set temples and heavy-bottom frame lines, will add width to that narrower part of your face. Avoid cat eye frames or frames with decorative temples, which is wide at the forehead, as it will draw attention to the wideness.

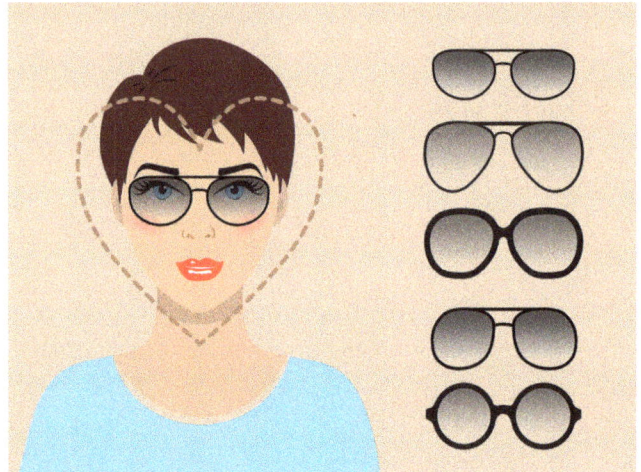

Round or square frames with curved edges will help draw attention away from a broad forehead.

Avoid frames with decorative temples or embellished tops that will draw attention to the broadness of the forehead.

Inverted Triangle Face Shape

The inverted triangle face shape is longer than it is wide, and the broadest part of the face is the forehead. This shape is similar to the heart shape, but the difference is that the hairline is straight and the forehead is a bit wider.

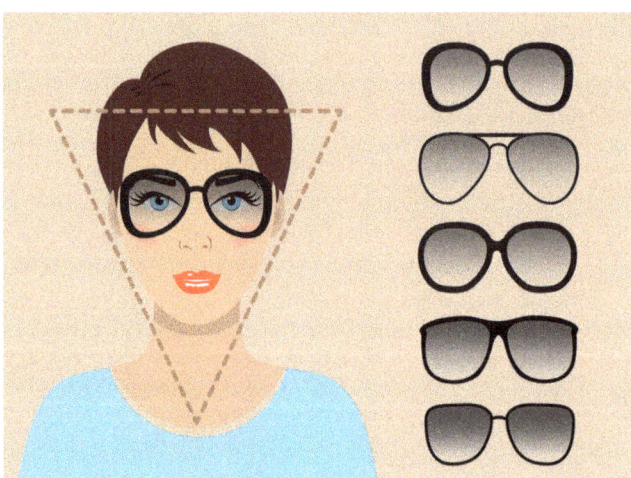

Round or square frames with curved edges will help draw attention away from a broad forehead.

Avoid frames with decorative temples or embellished tops and outstanding colours that will draw attention to the broad forehead.

Triangle Face Shape

A triangle face shape is longer than it is wide. The forehead is considerably narrower than the jawline, and the chin is square and noticeably flat in shape. Add width with heavily accented frames to emphasize the narrow upper third of the face. You can achieve accentuation through colour and detailing on the top half of the frame or through cat eye shapes.

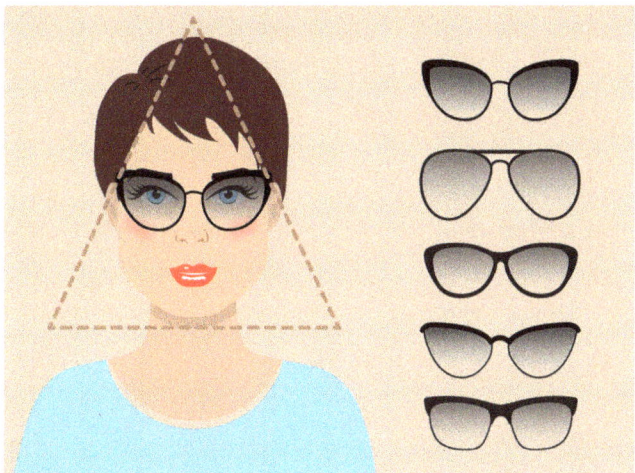

Frames that suit a triangle face are the butterfly, cat eye, flat top, and aviator shapes.

Avoid square and narrow frame styles that have more width than depth, and narrow ovals. It will draw attention to the large jawline.

Rectangle Face Shape

The rectangle face is longer than it is wide. Forehead and jawline are similar width in appearance. Cheeks and the sides of the face are straight. The forehead is broad and most likely straight around the hairline, with a noticeable square and/or flat chin.

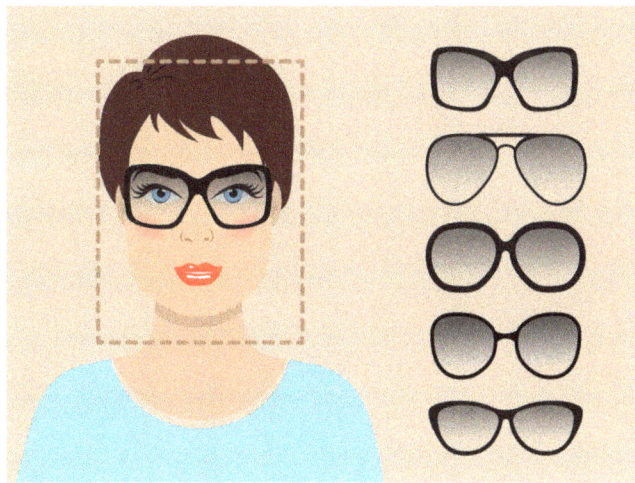

Wear larger frame styles that have soft edges. The larger frames will give the illusion of extra face width and break up the length of the face. Aviator frames will work as well.

Avoid squares, narrow ovals, and rectangular frames.

Round Face Shape

This face has curved lines, and the width and length are approximately the same width. The chin is round in shape with no hard lines. To make a round face appear thinner and longer, wear rectangle frames. Depending on the fashion, you can also wear squarish and roundish frames where the outer corners are lifted. A round face is similar to the square face but with round corners, that is why true square- and round frames will draw attention to the roundness of the face.

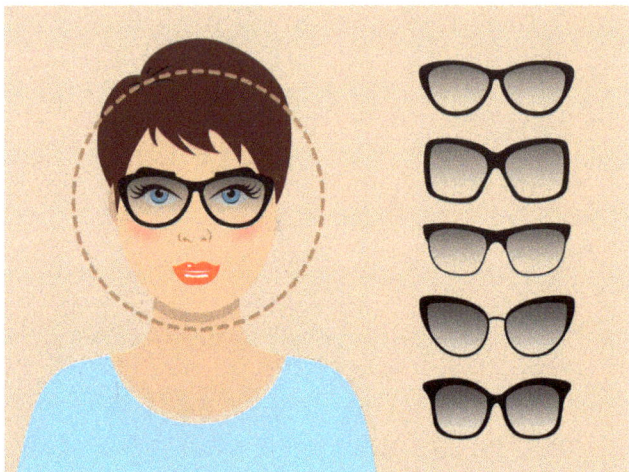

Rectangular frame shapes are a great choice because it will break the roundness. Round and square shapes with a slight lift on top corners are better.

Avoid true square and round frames.

Washing and Caring for Your Clothes

The Best Washing and Caring Techniques for Your Clothes

Fashion can be an investment, and every investment needs to come with proper maintenance. Proper caring techniques will extend the lifetime of your clothes, especially the pieces that you have spent more on. It is important not to over-wash your clothes either, because the colours fade quicker and the fabric structure changes. The lifetime of quality garments can be expanded to ten years or longer if properly cared for. When you can stretch the years of wearing your clothes, you will save money which can be used towards a special gift, like jewellery, shoes, spa treatments, or maybe enjoying a nice holiday every now and then. On the other hand, you can build up your wardrobe. You will also look professional at all times, and people will notice you when your clothes appear in good shape and colour.

Clothing care labels are required on garments by law in many countries. Sometimes instructions are typed out in words; otherwise, you will notice different symbols known as pictograms. They are usually an insert attached on the inside of the garment, somewhere on the side and closer to the hemline of a shirt, jacket, or skirt. For trousers, it is usually on the inside, under the waistband. A lot of people are not aware of them, and some decide to ignore them. Others have no clue what it means. They are an important part of ensuring that your garment is treated properly when laundering, ironing, and drying, to prolong its useful life.

There are different labelling schemes in different countries, and hopefully, there can be a generalized shift to international labelling. It is important to know that if a symbol indicates washing in hot water and tumble-drying, washing in cold water and drying on a clothes-line are also acceptable, as long as you do not use harsher methods than the instructions. The preferred washing and drying methods are cold to low water temperature, a low spinning cycle to reduce wrinkles, and line–drying in the shade, away from direct sunlight, to prolong the colours and shape of clothes.

The following are explanations of the most common home laundering and dry-cleaning symbols or pictograms you'll find as a care label inside each garment. If there are no instructions in a garment, it may be external instructions in the form of attached pricing and labelling to the garment.

Washing Pictograms		Drying Pictograms	
	Machine-wash through the use of warmest available water, detergent, or soap, and agitation.		Hang to dry, can be in sun or shade.
	Machine-wash with permanent press. Regular cycle, but use the slow spin of the delicate cycle to reduce wrinkles.		Drip-dry. Do no spin or wring the garment before hanging.
	Machine wash, gentle or delicate. Slow wash cycle and slow spin cycle. Reduce time.		Flat-dry on portable clothes drying rack to prevent garment from stretching while drying.
	Hand-wash with water, detergent, or soap, with gentle hand manipulation.		Dry in the shade to prevent colours from fading quickly.
	Do–not–wash symbol, usually accompanied by dry–clean only symbol.		Do not dry, usually accompanied by dry-clean only.
	Water temperature should not exceed thirty degrees or whatever temperature is showing in the tub symbol.		Dry–clean. With any solvent, any cycle, any moisture, any heat.
	Do not wring the clothes after handwashing.		Do not dry-clean. It is usually accompanied by another washing method.

Tumble-Dry Pictograms		Ironing Pictograms	
▢◯	*Tumble-dry-Normal.* May be tumble-dried regularly at hottest available setting.	(iron)	Regular ironing may be performed at any temperature, steam or dry.
▢◉	*Tumble-dry-Normal. Low Heat.* May be regularly tumble-dried on a low heat setting.	(iron with one dot)	Regular ironing may be performed at *low temperature* setting, steam or dry.
▢⊙⊙	*Tumble-dry-Normal. Medium heat.* May be regularly tumble-dried on a medium heat setting.	(iron with two dots)	Regular ironing may be performed at *medium temperature* setting, steam or dry.
▢⋯	*Tumble-dry-Normal. High heat.* May be regularly tumble-dried on a high heat setting.	(iron with three dots)	Regular ironing may be performed at *high temperature* setting, steam or dry.
▢●	*Tumble-dry-Normal. No heat.* May be regularly tumble-dried only at no-heat or air-only setting.	(iron with X)	*Do not iron.* Item may not be smoothed or finished with an iron.
▢◯ (with line)	*One line:* tumble-dry, permanent press, medium heat and cool-down cycle. *Two lines:* tumble-dry only on gentle setting.	(iron with lines under)	*Do not steam.* Steam may harm the garment; dry ironing is acceptable at indicated temperature.
▢⊗	*Do not tumble-dry;* usually accompanied by another drying method.	(iron with dot and lines under)	Iron, no steam.

166

Bleaching Pictograms	
△	Bleach when needed. Any commercial bleach product may be used in the laundering process.
⚠ (triangle with X)	Do not bleach. No bleach product may be used. The garment is not colourfast or structurally able.
△ (striped)	Non-chlorine bleach only when needed. Chlorine bleach may not be used.
⚠ (striped triangle with X)	No chlorine bleach may be used but non-chlorinebleach if needed.
Ⓐ	Dry-clean with any solvent. This is usually used with other restrictions on proper dry-cleaning procedures.
Ⓕ	Dry-clean using only petroleum solvent. This is usually used with other restrictions.
Ⓟ	Any dry-cleaning solvent other than trichloroethylene may be safely used.

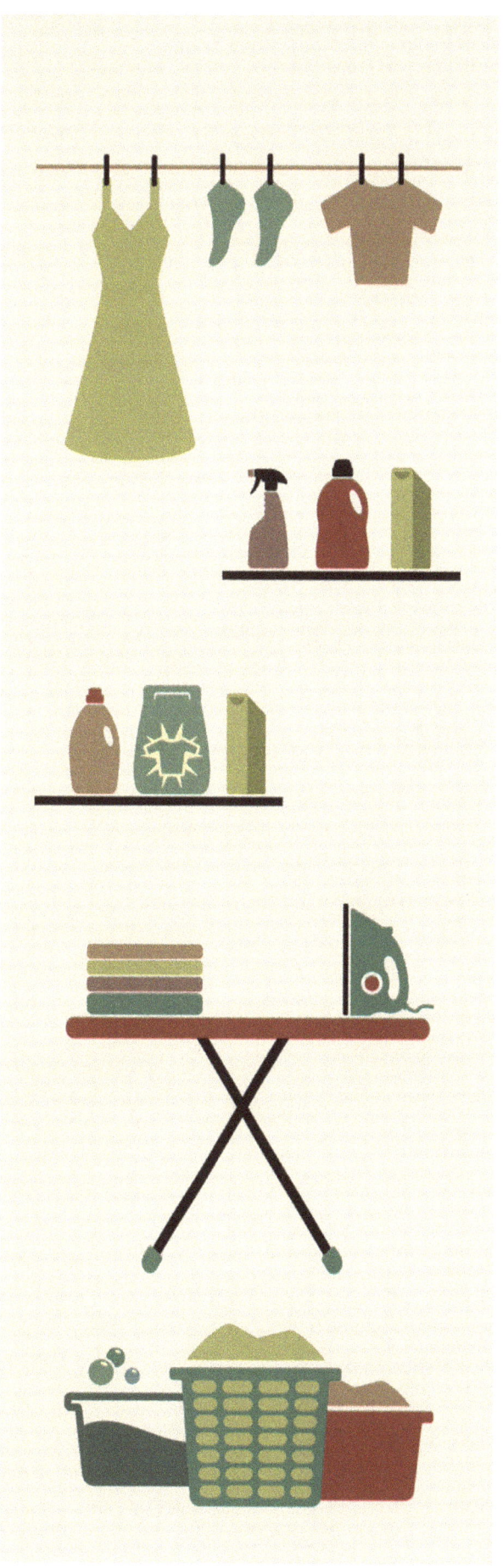

167

Many washing machines these days have a control dial to choose your wash. There are a lot of different dial settings, which range from woollens to heavy-duty wash. From hot- to cold-water settings, some even have a degree setting to choose the exact water temperature for the wash. We are very fortunate to have the luxury of washing machines and all the high-technology features. Just think how difficult it must have been with no washing machines or equipment in earlier years.

The earliest special-purpose mechanical washing device, before washing machines, was the washboard that was invented in 1797 by Nathaniel Briggs of New Hampshire. By the mid- 1850s, steam-driven commercial laundry machinery were on sale in the UK and US. The rotary washing machine for home use was patented by Hamilton Smith in 1858. Electricity was not commonly available until at least 1930. Some early washing machines were operated by a low-speed, single-cylinder, hit-and-miss gasoline engine. The first domestic automatic washing machine was introduced in 1937. In the world today, there are still people who have to hand-wash their clothes. The first washing tool created, the washboard, is a luxury for them. If you own an automatic washing machine, consider yourself very privileged.

Let's all be water conscious though by only using the water level required for the size of clothing load. Do not allow the water level to fill up the whole tub, at extra-large water level, where clothes only fill up to half of the machine tub. A lot of machines have an eco-wash sensor setting, and will only fill up the tub to the level of clothes.

Washing your clothes to the correct laundering instructions are important, but the main reasons why we have to wash our clothes regularly is to get rid of sweat, dead skin, and skin oils. Shirts, bras, underwear, and camisoles that sit close to our genital area, breasts, or armpits cannot be worn for two full consecutive days, as bacterial invasion may hit the second day with an undesirable smell. Women need to be very careful because they may not realize it themselves, but other people will get the bad odour first before they do. It is as if the wearer gets used to the smell, and they do not realize how bad the smell is.

First and foremost, women have an obligation to their family, friends, colleagues, husband, and the public around them to make sure their clothes are without any stains or bad odour.

One bad stain is make-up stain on the clothes of women who wear excessive amounts of foundation. Perfect style cannot overcome stains and bad odour due to sweating or wearing the same underwear and clothes without regular washing or dry-cleaning. The other bad habit is the overuse of perfume on garments that really need a wash to get rid of the odour. Every woman must have come across at least one incident during their lifetime, where another woman was so smelly, that they had to close their airways and gasp for air after the woman moved out of their smelling range. Of course, the same count for all the men out there, and it is our duty to train them well. Most women will have a brother, a husband, or a son at some point in their lives. Let's make an effort to train the men in our lives well.

I honestly believe there is no ugly person on this earth. The only problem is that some never had the opportunity to be educated in style to understand how to look their best. Another unfortunate cause is that some do not love themselves because of different scenarios in their life.

Fabrics that need special care when washing: wool, cotton, silk, lingerie, linen, jersey material, lace, bras, any fabric with metallic thread.

Clothes and fabrics that need to be hand-washed and drip dried for the best results and an extended lifetime: Clothes with the hand-wash only pictogram, lingerie, bras, silk, chiffon, and garments made with lace fabrics. Alternatively, you can use a mesh laundry bag in the machine to protect them during the wash cycle.

Fabrics That Can Be Put through the Tumble Dryer

Tumble-dry garments only when garments have the symbol in the care label. When it says 'Do not tumble-dry', follow the instructions carefully; otherwise, you run the risk of wrecking the garment.

A great trick is to put bed linen and cotton shirts in the tumble dryer for five minutes before you hang it out to dry. This will get rid of most creases and make ironing easier and faster.

Towels can also be put in the tumble dryer for five minutes after they have dried on the line to make it feel softer.

The Best Ways to Hang Your Washing to Dry

Turn all shirts and jackets upside down and hang each on a hanger. This will help the colours to last for longer.

A plastic or aluminium hanger is recommended because it is easier to slide the wet garments over. Turning all garments upside down when hanging will help keep the colours beautiful for longer. You can wrap elastic bands on each of the hanger's sides to prevent slippery garments from sliding off, or you can use pegs to secure the top bar of the hanger.

Ladies, there is another thing that I feel I have to mention. I came across a few women who were working in an office with me over the years who made comments like this when it was their turn to wash the office tea towels: 'I do not mind washing it because I have to run the washing machine anyway'.

This was a shock to my system to realize that they threw the office tea towels in the washing machine with the rest of their clothes. We as women cannot wash tea towels, which we use to dry cutlery and dishes with, along with our underwear and dirty clothes. Everything in the kitchen needs to be handled hygienically since it gets in contact with our food, plates, cups, pots, and utensils.

The following steps are fast and effective to hand-wash clothes and save on laundry soap and water:

Separate the white, light–coloured, and dark-coloured clothing.

Fill up the laundry tub with lukewarm water to the required level (depending on the load), and add laundry liquid.

It is recommended to use an earth choice laundry liquid, which is safe for the environment, and most importantly, safe to use on fabrics and will make the colours stay beautiful for longer.

Submerge the clothing and gently agitate the clothes for thirty seconds to one minute. Rub stained spots with a laundry block of soap and rub under the arms of shirts and necklines to get rid of the sweat and odour trapped in the fabric.

Also rub the seam line of the pants to remove any dirt that may have come from the ground or shoes.

Transfer your whites and light-coloured clothing bit by bit after each wash to a solid laundry basket, by lifting it out of the water and gently squeezing out as much water that you can without wringing it.

Use the same tub of water now to wash all your dark and black clothing in the same way as just mentioned. Transfer the dark and black clothing to another solid laundry basket that is separate from the whites. Keeping it separate will ensure that the black garments do not stain the whites.

Drain the sink, and refill with cool water and add a softener which is safe for the environment and safe on your clothing fabrics. Submerge all the whites and light-coloured clothing and rinse all by pushing each clothing piece up and down in the water until all remaining soap is removed. Also give the laundry basket a quick rinse to get rid of any soap before placing the clothes back after rinsing.

Gently squeeze the excess water from each garment and place back in the laundry bucket.

Do not twist or wring the clothes, as it may stretch the fibres and ruin the fabric. When the whites and light-coloured clothing are all rinsed, submerge all the dark and black clothing in the same sink with water and softener, and follow the same process.

Rinse the laundry basket quickly to get rid of any soap or coloured leftover water before placing the rinsed clothes back in the laundry basket.

Now you are ready to hang your clothes outside in the shade. If your clothes line is in direct sunlight, you can invest in a portable, folding clothes-drying rack that you can move to shading areas, such as next to your home.

Hang all shirts, jackets, and dresses on a hanger before hanging on the clothes line. You can stabilize each hanger by placing clothing pegs close to the hanger's hook on each side of the washing line. This technique will keep the garments apart so that all do not end up in a bundle on the line without any air space between each to dry.

The rest of the washing including trousers, skirts, socks, underwear, etc. can be hanged on the washing line or clothes-drying rack with pegs. It is recommended to turn your trousers and skirts upside down when you hang it outside on the washing line. This technique will prevent quick fading of the garment colours.

Where possible, always hang clothes in the shade out of direct sunlight.

Ironing Your Clothes

When you compare a lady whose clothes are all nicely ironed with someone who looks all wrinkly, you will realize why it is so important to iron your clothes. You will look so much more neat and professional. I bet you will even feel and look more stylish, because that is how I feel.

Seven Reasons Why Ironing Your Clothes Is Important

1. Your overall appearance will look neat and tidy.
2. Other people are attracted to neat and tidy individuals.
3. Ironing your clothes shows that you are taking pride in your appearance.
4. It saves you money rather than taking it to the dry-cleaners.
5. Clothes will last longer, as it will not come into contact with perchloroethylene, which is a harmful chemical used in dry-cleaning processes.
6. It is proven that ironed clothes make us feel less cloudy and more special.
7. Turning up for a job interview in a shirt obviously full of creases will decrease your chance of getting the job.

Of course, there are ways to handle certain garments that you do not need to iron. By following the next procedures, you will not need to iron T-shirts, jeans, PJs, and tracksuits.

After you have taken it off the washing line, put it through the tumble dryer on hot for three to five minutes. Make sure to check the care label of each garment before inserting them in the dryer. When you take it out of the tumble dryer, take it to your bed and lay each garment flat on the bed, while still warm, and stroke it with your hands as if you are ironing it. Put each garment on top of the other, and work your way quickly through the bundle before it cools down.

Wait till all the clothes have cooled down and then hang or fold them up before placing them in the drawer. Do not bundle them in a drawer after you have done so much to make it wrinkle-free. Keep it nicely folded to hold its smooth look.

To do an easy and good ironing job, you require *good tools*.

You need a good steam iron with built-in safety features, water spray bottle, press cloth, and a good, sturdy ironing board, the wider, the better. The surface should be smooth and without any folds. A cushioned surface produces the best results.

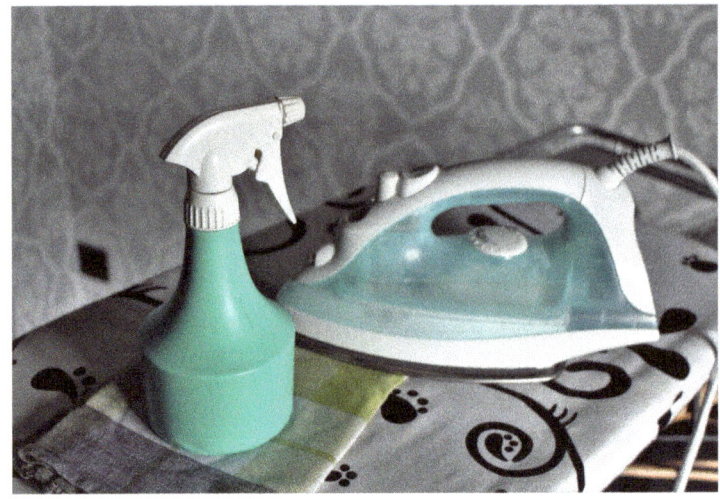

Ironing Tips

Iron thick fabrics on the inside first, then on the outside.

Spray wrinkled shirts lightly with water before ironing, it will get rid of the creases quicker and will produce a smoother finish.

Place a small to medium towel that is rolled inside a short- or long sleeved garment, when ironing. You'll just have to steam the sleeve then rather than flat ironing. This technique will prevent the crease you normally create with flat ironing.

Do not iron over buttons. Slip the point of the iron underneath each button.

Iron all delicate garments on the inside or with a press cloth to prevent burning or leaving shiny iron marks.

Pressing trousers and shirts is just what the word say. You press the iron on the fabric for one to two seconds, lift it up, and press again on the next spot that has not been pressed before. Pressing will not produce shiny marks or patches on a garment; whereas sliding movements with the iron can. A too hot iron can also cause shiny marks; especially on double fabrics like seamlines or pockets. Another safeguard is to always use a press cloth between the iron and the garment, which will protect the fabric from the direct hot plate of the iron. The best press cloth is the mesh guard type as shown in the picture.

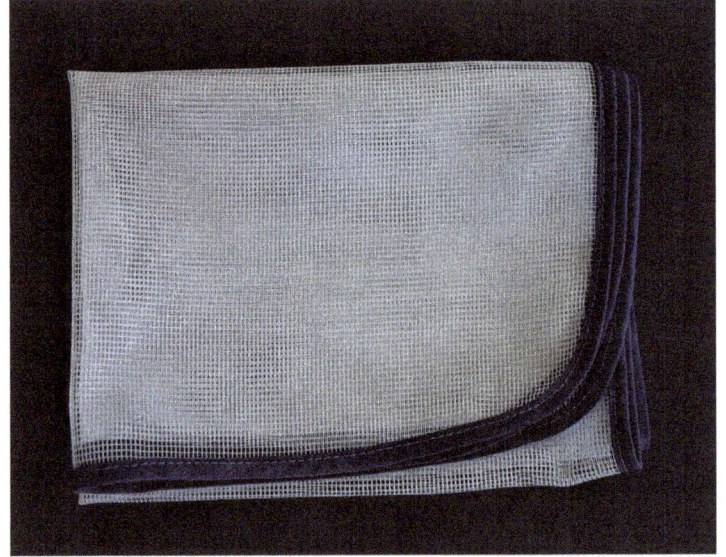

Hot ironing pressing cloth mesh guard.

The Best Ironing Sequence

Read the labels first to determine if garment can be ironed and the instructed temperature.

If you're unsure what the temperature of the iron should be, start with a low setting and increase it till you reach the correct temperature that removes the creases.

Corporate Shirts with Collars

1. For a shirt with many wrinkles, spray it lightly with water before ironing.

2. Start with the collar by pressing the iron in the centre of the wrong side of the collar, and work your way to the edges. Now flip the collar back and turn it around so that the inside of the collar is on top, which is the back of the neck. Give one press and hold it for two to three seconds. Do not press the edges; it should have a slight lift.

3. Drape one side of the shirt's panels over the ironing board, and work your way to the back and other side panel.

4. Place one sleeve on the ironing board and flatten all fabric with your hands first. Iron each side of the sleeve. To prevent too many wrinkles where the cuff joins the sleeve, insert a rolled-up towel inside the shirt when ironing the bottom half of the sleeve.

5. Drape one side of the shirt's shoulder over the edge of the iron board and press with the iron from the shoulder to the back. It's also called the yoke. Repeat on the other side.

6. Some fabrics may have made small wrinkles on the front and back panels again as you worked your way through. You can quickly just press any wrinkles if necessary.

7. Hang the shirt on a hanger straight after to prevent it from forming new wrinkles when you just lay it down. To save time, have a clothing rail next to you to hang each shirt straight after ironing, or hang it in the wardrobe.

Trousers

1. If the trousers have pockets, turn them inside out and iron the pockets first. Then turn them back.

2. For those with no pockets, just start with this step. Pull the waistband of the trousers over the edge of the iron board and press (not stroke) each panel under the waistband.

3. When done with all panels under the waistband, lay the trousers flat on the iron board, with one leg lying on top of the other and with the joined lines in the centre

of the leg. Make sure to smooth all the lines with your hands first before pressing (not stroking).

4. Press from the top to the bottom, lift the top leg up, and press the bottom leg, which is the inside of the other leg. Then flip the trousers to repeat on the other side.

5. Lay the trousers flat on the bed, couch, or table to cool down before hanging it on a hanger. This will prevent a fold halfway down the legs.

Dresses

1. If the dress fabric is cotton with a lot of wrinkles, lightly spray the whole dress with water before starting to iron.

2. Iron dresses from the collar down. Use a press cloth to prevent any shiny marks.

3. Pull the bodice over the edge of the iron board and press each panel.

4. Now press the sleeves, if any, one at a time, first the one side then turning to press the other side. Use a rolled-up towel in the sleeves before ironing if you do not want a definite crease from the shoulder down.

5. Move on to the skirt part of the dress. First, turn the dress inside out and iron the skirt part in the inside. Pull one side over the edge of the iron board and work your way through the whole skirt.

6. Turn the dress back and hang it straight after it's been ironed.

Skirts

1. Turn the skirt inside out first.

2. Pull the skirt over the free edge of the iron board. Iron each section and work your way around.

3. If it has a slip, iron the slip after you ironed the skirt, but make sure the temperature is not to warm. Or use a press cloth to protect it from producing a shiny iron mark.

4. Remove the skirt from the iron board; turn it back with the right side up.

5. Place the waistband flat on the iron board, place a press cloth over it, and start pressing. Flip it around and repeat on the other side.

6. Place it on a flat surface till you are done with all your ironing before you hang it, or hang it straight away.

Building Your Self-Confidence

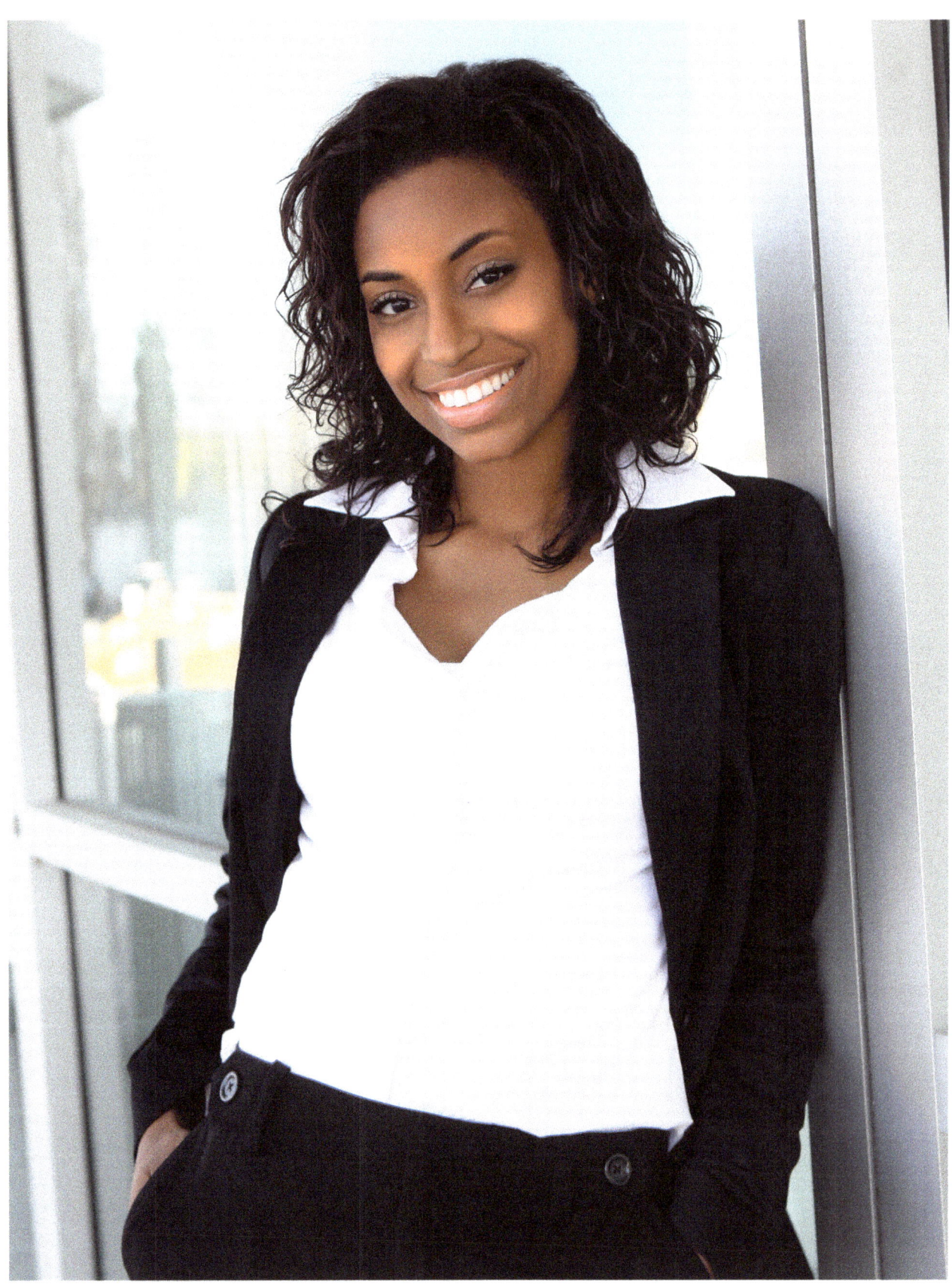

What is Self-Confidence?

Self-confidence is made up of what you are feeling, what you are thinking, what you know, and what your opinion is of yourself. Accepting what you are and not wanting to be like someone else, but working towards the best version of yourself that you can be. Overcome your failures and try again. Confidence in oneself is very necessary to succeed in all of life's challenges. When confidence steps in, fear steps out. The fear of failing and what others will think of you. And yes, I am definitely not meaning that you can go out to hurt, trick, and steal and not worry what others think of you. Always operate and live your life with a good character.

Good character includes all the aspects of a person's behaviour and attitude that make up that person's personality. The qualities of having a good character are to be honest in all your dealings, be a person of integrity at all times, have a generous spirit, treat others with respect, have an attitude of gratitude in life, be trustworthy, not live a life of self-gain only, be self-disciplined, have self-control, not be self-absorbed, be fair in everything and to everyone, not steal, not hurt someone intentionally, not being afraid to fail, not having an attitude that the world owes you something and you do not have to do your part, and to have compassion for others.

There are two types of confident people:

1. Those who are so confident in themselves, that you immediately feel inferior in their presence. They come across as arrogant, and you feel uncomfortable in their presence. They keep telling you about their successes and how good they are.

2. The second type of person is confident, and it almost feels as if their confidence rubs off on you. You instantly feel more confident in their presence. You enjoy being around them. This person will always compliment you and try to make you look better. They do not rub all their accomplishments under your nose all the time.

Strive to be a person where your confidence rubs off on others, where you help others gain confidence rather than make them feel worthless in your presence. Sometimes others just need encouragement from that one person to make a difference in their lives.

With confidence and love, we can reach out to the people around us and the people we meet for the first time.

There's no doubt that self-confidence is very important to succeed in all of life's challenges, but so many people struggle to find theirs. Many talk about self-confidence, but there are no clear instructions to follow on how to gain it. Self-confidence is an 'inner-self' thing, and different elements and events during a person's life, help to birth self-confidence. Some people take years to gain their self-confidence, while others discover it as a child.

We as women play a huge role in our children's lives. Some of you reading this book are already a mother or grandmother, and some of you are mothers-to-be sometime in the future.

The Merriam-Webster Dictionary describes *self-confidence* as 'confidence in oneself and in one's powers and abilities'.

The phrases 'You cannot do it', 'It is not possible', 'There is no way that you'll be able to do it' or 'Watch out, you are going to hurt yourself' are all too familiar. As children, we have heard it so many times from our parents, from our siblings, from our teachers, from our family members, from our friends, and from others. All these fears and doubts have infiltrated our mind and being; therefore, we have to re-programme our minds with positive data that will make us more confident. Fill your mind with good thoughts like 'Yes, I can! It does not matter if I fail', 'I just have to try again another way', 'There is always a way, I just have to find it'.

As an inventor, Thomas Edison made 1,000 unsuccessful attempts at inventing the light bulb. A reporter asked him, 'How did it feel to fail 1,000 times?'. And Edison replied, 'I didn't fail 1,000 times. The light bulb was an invention with 1,000 steps'.

Arthur Ashe said, 'One important key to success is self-confidence. An important key to self-confidence is preparation'. Since we are born, our self-confidence will start to grow. A baby cannot automatically be born as an already self-confident being. Each of us is born with a certain personality that can help us be more confident. Our parents are the most important people in our life to help us gain confidence. The way we are being brought up determines our confidence early in life. The second most important people in our life are our grandparents then our school-teachers, followed by our family and friends, all the people around us during the day, even the people we meet for the first time.

The most amazing truth is that we do not have to let our past determine our confidence level and future. Although we had people in our life influencing us to a certain point, we have the power in us to change our way of thinking and what we think of ourselves. Do not delay! Today is the day where you say to yourself, 'I am beautiful, intelligent, and confident. My future looks bright and successful. I am looking forward to my wonderful future'. Say it to yourself every day, and see how your life transforms.

The first thing you have to do in order to improve your mind is, to take control of your thoughts during the day and recognise when your thoughts are negative and fearful. As soon as you identified negativity, consciously move your thoughts to happy memories and positive thoughts. Our brain is constantly forming new connections and moulding itself into how we are telling it to operate, and is therefore highly re-programmable at any age. So the power is in our hands to change our lives by feeding our brain with happy and positive thoughts. Earl Nightingale said: 'Whatever we plant in our subconscious mind and nourish with repetition and emotion will one day become a reality'.

Dealing with Bullying

Bullying affects our self-confidence. People around us have all different issues and hurts that they have to carry at different stages in their life. Sometimes when we are so happy, we have to withstand bad attitudes, hurtful words, and actions from others. Our confidence level will determine how we will deal with it. Parents and their children also hurt one another sometimes. It can be consciously or unconsciously.

Unfortunately, some people hurt others because it has become a habit, and they show no mercy or guilt over what they do to others. These master bullies usually think they are always right and the other person or people are always wrong. When someone say something that hurts you and you know it is not true, do not even give a second thought to it. Those second and continuous thoughts that we give to things said to us unfairly will start to grow on us, and we'll start to wonder if maybe we are as they say. Let me tell you, when you pamper all the ugly and damning words spoken to you, you will just waste valuable time in your life. Rather, spend the time reading and listening to positive materials such as books or videos. Go to seminars that will increase your knowledge and confidence in who you are. Knowledge is power, and it builds a person's character. The more general knowledge we have, the more confident we feel in life.

I think mothers of all teenagers and young adults have to endure a lot of physical and verbal bullying from their children. On the other hand, it is not undeniable that there is an enormous amount of children suffering from abuse by their parents or other people or children. Being bullied or bullying others is not cool, and we have to stop it as soon as we can.

The different types of bullying are verbal, physical, and cyber.

Verbal bullying is when someone uses words in a negative way, such as insults and words to put you down. The overall goal of a verbal bully is to cause another person to feel worthless by attacking their self-esteem. They will say something to you to hurt you, or lower your self-esteem. Do not be afraid to stand up for yourself and be assertive, but avoid being argumentative. Most verbal bullies have a low self-esteem, and therefore, they feel they need to make themselves look good by attacking others verbally. But they mostly hide their insecurities by coming across as overly confident. They usually are very popular, and others do not want to stand up to them in the fear of being bullied themselves. A verbal bully wants to manipulate and control a person.

How do you stop verbal bullying against you?

Let the verbal bully know that their attitude and behaviour are unacceptable. Tell them calmly to stop bullying you. Say, 'That is enough, don't talk to me that way'. You can also ask the bully why they feel that way. This will give them a chance to tell you their reasons for wanting to hurt you with negative and hurtful words. It may be a good way to talk it out and stop the verbal bullying against you from that person forever.

When it comes to *physical bullying*, it is never acceptable, and you must not be afraid to seek help. Tell someone immediately. Physical bullies may threaten you with more harm if you tell someone. In this case, find a safe haven for you to stay while telling someone in an authority position; this will help you to stop the physical bullying against you. No matter what the reason is for the bully to think he or she can physical harm you, it is never all right. Being aware of physical bullying against another and not doing anything about it, makes you just as guilty. If every person in this world is speaking up against physical bullying, we will make this world a better place.

These are the reasons why people think they have the right to physically bully others: religious views, religious discrimination, misogynous views, discriminating views, sexism, child abuse, or any other unfair reason.

If you are a woman or child trapped in any of the above bullying acts, get out as soon as you can. God has made you to be someone special, and you do not deserve being treated this way. Get help as soon as possible to help relieve you from this unfair act.

Be mindful that your words and actions do not provoke being bullied. You cannot point the finger at the other person bullying you if it starts with you. If a woman yells at her husband, boyfriend, or any other person every day, it can make them lose control.

Cyber-bullying can be just as detrimental for someone. If you are getting bullied via social media networks, it is best to ignore it and not to get involved in cyber-bullying yourself. In the case where you feel it is too much to handle and the words said are making you feel worthless, cancel your account and get off social media as soon as possible. Rather, communicate with people who have a positive influence in your life. Get around people who compliment you and who lift you up rather than breaking you off via the words they say. As already mentioned, do not let their words get to you. Forget about it and focus on other positive things in life.

No person on this earth deserves to be bullied via physical actions or words. If you see someone else getting bullied, stand up for them; they may need someone to stand up for them to realize that what they're going through is not right. Your actions may give them the courage to stand up and get out of the bullying act. Under no circumstances should you get involved in any physical actions though. Just say in a calm voice to the bully that what you have just seen and experienced from them is not right and very disappointing. Make sure to leave and stay out of any confrontation.

You must have experienced the following while driving or being a passenger in a car: someone cuts in between you and the car in front of you. It is shocking to see how they think they can do this without the desired space between your car and theirs. This act usually causes you to slam on your brakes to make sure you do not smash into them. This kind of action on the road shows me that the person driving the car is as bombastic and most likely a bully in life because they do not care about the other person, as long as they get their way. I remember when I taught my kids to drive. I said to them, 'In cases where you missed your turn-off, do not just cut right in front of another car and cause a possible crash. You just have to drive around the block again and make sure you are in the right lane when you come closer to your turn-off the next time.' In everything you do in life, try your best not to cause a problem for others even when it comes to driving on the road.

Healthy Relationships

A family shares strong emotional bonds and common values, goals, and responsibilities. Family members contribute significantly to the well-being of each other. Healthy family relationships help all members of the family to feel safe and connected to one another. Of course, there are some times conflict between family members, which is a normal part of family life. Conflicts can occur between adults, between children, or between adults and children. Examples of healthy conflicts could be disagreements about household chores, parenting decisions, house rules, siblings not wanting to share toys, or siblings wanting to watch television.

All families have times when tempers flare, feelings get hurt, and misunderstandings occur. The important fact here is how we deal with it. Violence is never the answer. Issues and feelings need to be discussed in a civil manner and, if not resolved, seek the help of a professional. There is no shame in it when families need the help of a professional every now and then. They are qualified to help individuals and families with issues. Occasionally, it is hard to get children to go with the parents to a professional. Mothers, I would suggest then that you go by yourself so that the professional advises you how best to deal with a situation.

Families that overcome differences and stick together no matter what, can achieve great success on all levels in life. A healthy family is created when members put family first.

Unhealthy relationships are defined as relationships in which physical, sexual, psychological, or emotional violence take place. These kinds of relationships are filled with negativity and bring out the worst in people rather than the best. It is serious, and these acts need to be stopped at all cost.

Mothers are very important role models for their children, and when they get mistreated by their dads or whoever in life, we as mothers need to protect them. When a mother has tried everything and still cannot protect her children from violence, it has become time to speak up and talk to the authorities.

Another sad fact I want to bring attention to is the fact that there are a lot of mothers who get bullied by their children. Do not allow it! If you do everything in your power to be good to your child and they are still mistreating you, get help! As a mother, you do not deserve to be treated with disrespect and violence.

A few years ago, I went shopping and saw a woman in her late teens or early twenties who was shouting and insulting her dad all the way as they were walking from the car park to the shopping centre. At the time, I was so shocked and did not say anything. I have never seen this kind of act in public and was wondering how she must treat him at home if she does that to him in town in front of spectators. He looked like a person with low self-confidence. That is usually what happens to an individual who does not have enough self-confidence; others think they can treat them with disrespect. I would like to take this opportunity to let all mothers know that you must not take any abusive treatment from your adult children. If you have an abusive child who is of working age, let them go and grow up before they can come and live under your roof again.

I also found that parents are very ashamed to talk about their problems with their children to others. They would rather pretend as if everything is hunky-dory. Usually, they feel it is a reflection on them and feel responsible for their children's actions. When you as a mother can say with assurance that you have done the best you can to bring up your children, all you can do is pray for them. And when they move out of your home, do not lock yourself up and not get out there to make friends. This is the best time for you to catch-up with friends and make new ones. Be happy and friendly in life because these positive characteristics attract positive people and situations.

When it comes to friends also, choose them with caution. You should have friends who compliment you and who uplift you. A good friend is someone you can trust, someone who is loyal, honest, non-judgmental, and cares about you. Your friends will have a big influence on how you think, feel, and behave. Do not worry if you lose some friends along the way. You'll find that you have different friends during the different seasons in your life. As a person grows in knowledge and skills, it may be that you get bored with your current friends. The actual fact is that your interests have changed, and that is why you will constantly try to find like-minded people around you. Like-minded people inspire each other and contribute greatly to one another's success. Find friends who are interested in you as a person and who wants you to succeed. The right friends will make you more confident.

Easy Steps to Help You Gain Your Self-Confidence

- Start loving and accepting yourself. Do not try to change your look to look like someone else. Groom yourself to be the best version of yourself.
- Start loving others. The characteristics of love are explained on the next page.
- See how you can add value to other people's lives.
- Look at yourself and decide which areas you would like to improve on. Is it your appearance, knowledge, or spiritual level?
- Put things in action to work towards your goals, and do not delay.

- Our appearance and grooming have a direct link to our self-confidence. So work on your appearance and make sure you are well-groomed every day, and your self-confidence will grow by a huge step.
- Do not believe any negative thoughts telling you that you are not good enough. If someone is saying something to you which hurt, let it slide off you. Speak good and positive things out loud to yourself every day. Researchers have shown that these tactics really change people's minds and they become more positive and confident.
- For definite success in reaching your goals and becoming more confident, start writing it down in a journal.
- Build your knowledge every day through reading books, researching information, watching educational videos, and furthering your studies. Have a goal to learn something new every day, even if it is just a new word and its meaning you did not know before.
- A person is never too old to learn. Enrol in a study course regularly, and work your way slowly through to complete it. Someone who does not grow daily will fall behind and later even move backwards. The world is constantly changing, and we will have to grow with it in order to keep our confidence. By keeping your brain active, you will stay younger for longer, and you will for sure build your self-confidence.
- Have an attitude of gratitude in life for what you have and who helps you.

Characteristics of Love

Showing love is not all about intimate relationships; it is so much more. To love someone is to operate in the following characteristics:

- *Love is patient*: being able to accept or tolerate delays, problems, or suffering without becoming annoyed or angry.
- *Love is kind:* having a helpful and sympathetic nature or personality.
- *Love does not envy:* not being jealous of the other person.
- *Love does not boast:* no bragging or self-praise.
- *Love is not proud:* having excessively high opinion of oneself or one's importance.
- *Love does not dishonour others:* will bring no shame or disgrace to other people.
- *Love is not self-seeking:* only caring about yourself.
- *Love is not easily angered:* not getting angry quickly.
- *Love keeps no record of wrongs:* forgiving people who have done you wrong.
- *Love does not delight in evil but rejoices with the truth:* not enjoying wrongdoings and disgraceful things against another.
- *Love always protects:* it means to keep a person safe from harm or injury.

- *Love always trusts:* all relationships must be built on trust.
- *Love always hopes:* a feeling of expectation and desire for something good to happen.
- *Love always perseveres:* keep going even in the face of difficulty or with little or no indication of success.

Source: Characteristics of Love, The Bible, 1 Corinthians 13:4-7

Final Note...

Not one person in the world has exactly the same gifts, talents, background, or future.

Do not try to be like someone else, because you will fail for sure.

Be the best version of yourself and the person God has created you to be.

Follow the dreams in your heart, and put the effort in to achieve them.

My Quick Reference Guide

This book belongs to: _____

Date: _____

My wrist measurement is: ☐ Small Scale   ☐ Medium Scale   ☐ Large Scale
(refer to page 32)

My body shape is: _____
(refer to pages 34-35)

My Style Personality is: _____
(refer to page 37-38)

Garment lines that I can wear successfully:
(refer to pages 40, 46, 47)

☐ Vertical Lines   ☐ Horizontal Lines   ☐ Diagonal Lines

My face shape is: _____
(refer to pages 49-52)

The best necklines for me:
(refer to pages 54-69)

_____   _____

_____   _____

_____   _____

_____   _____

The best shoulder lines for me:
(refer to pages 71-75)

_____   _____

_____   _____

_____   _____

_____   _____

I want to create optical illusion for these body parts:
(refer to pages 76-83)

	Body Part	Want to Achieve	How?
Examples	- Arms - Upper body - Bottom & thighs	- To look a bit shorter. - To look shorter. - To look smaller.	- Wear long sleeves with a cuff. - Wear horizontal lines, belt above middle line, V-neckline. - Wear vertical lines, straight knee length skirts, dark coloured skirts.

My body shape is: _____
(refer to pages 86-101)

The best styles for my body shape is on this page: _____

The Best Styles For Me

My skin undertone is:
(refer to pages 118-119)

☐ COOL   ☐ WARM   ☐ NEUTRAL

My colour season is: _____
(refer to pages 119-121)

My season colours to wear are on page _____
(refer to pages 122-125)

I flow between colour seasons:

My dominant characteristics are (refer to page 127) _____

_____

My secondary characteristic is (refer to page 128) _____

_____

Refer to the *Flow Seasonal Table* to find your flow season (on page 128).
My flow season is:

_____

My flow season colours to wear are on page: _____

My best colour jewellery to wear is: _____

The best frames for my face shape are:
(refer to pages 158-162)

_____   _____

_____   _____

_____   _____

I have made a decision today that I will love myself, and I am going to follow the next steps to build my self-confidence: (refer to pages 177-184)

Date: _____   Signed _____

_____

_____

_____

_____

_____

_____

_____

Bibliography

Breslau, Ellen, *'5 Reasons Your Body Shape Changes As You Age'*, <http://www.huffingtonpost.com/entry/5-reasons-your-body-shape-changes-as-you-age_us_55a808cbe4b0896514d0b2c7>accessed 18 March 2017.

Vernelen, Anja, *'Twelve Season Color Analysis'*, [website] <https://www.colormepretty.co/categories-2/12-season-color-analysis/, *What lead to the creation of the twelve season color analysis?*> accessed 20 March 2017.

WIKIPEDIA The Free Encyclopedia, *'Munsell color system'*, [website], <https://en.wikipedia.org/wiki/Munsell_color_system> accessed 25 March 2017.

Vision Service Plan, 'Glasses & Sunglasses Frames', [website] <https://www.vsp.com/how-to-choose-glasses.html?site_preference=SMARTPHONE> accessed 5 June 2017.

Morgan, Erinn, *'How To Choose The Best Eyeglasses For Your Face Shape And Coloring'*, http://www.allaboutvision.com/eyeglasses/eyeglasses_shape_color_analysis.htm> accessed 5 June 2017.

Liddelow, Jane, *'Assess Your Body Scale'*, [website] <http://www.style-makeover-hq.com/body-scale.html> accessed 6 June 2017.

Gorgeautiful.com, Fashion Tips and Tricks of All Time, *'Knowing the Right Necklines for Your Face and Body Shape (Part 1)'*, http://www.gorgeautiful.com/knowing-the-right-necklines-for-your-face-and-body-shape-part-1/> accessed 10 June 2017.

Jackson, C. *Color Me Beautiful, Discover Your Natural Beauty through Colours That Make You Look Great and Feel Fabulous* (Washington D.C. Acropolis Books Ltd, 1980), 77-79 and 83-93.

Jedinak, Arianna, 'Overview on the body shapes', [website] <http://www.joyofclothes.com/style-advice/shape-guides/the-rectangle.php> accessed 11 July 2017.

'But They Did Not Give Up', [website] <https://www.uky.edu/~eushe2/Pajares/OnFailingG.html> accessed 25 July 2017.

wikiHow, *'How to Deal With Verbal Bullying'*, [website] <https://www.wikihow.com/Deal-With-Verbal-Bullying> accessed 15 July 2017.

NIV Essentials Study Bible, *'Love Is Indispensable - 1 Corinthians 13 verses 4-7'*, (by Zondervan 2013),1449.

Shutterstock Images used in this book:

Indira's work, *'Sexy brunette woman skinny business style dress black color perfect body shape diet busy glamour lady casual style secretary diplomatic protocol office uniform stewardess air hostess etiquette suit - Stock photo ID: 488607823'*, Digital Image, < > accessed 28 November 2017.

Sermek, Gordana, *'Stripped female blouse isolated on white - Stock photo ID: 66739090'*, Digital Image, <https://www.shutterstock.com/image-photo/stripped-female-blouse-isolated-on- white-66739090?src=library> accessed 28 November 2017.

elenovsky, *'stripped sweater - Stock photo ID: 318944150'*, Digital Image, <https://www.shutterstock.com/image-photo/stripped-sweater-318944150?src=library> accessed 28 November 2017.

elenovsky, *'Stripped skirt - Stock photo ID: 438455407'*, Digital Image, <https://www.shutterstock.com/image-photo/stripped-skirt-438455407?src=library> accessed 28 November 2017.

maffi, *'black dress isolated on white background - Stock photo ID: 533351728'*, Digital Image, <https://www.shutterstock.com/image-photo/black-dress-isolated-on-white-background- 533351728?src=library> accessed 28 November 2017.

hifashion, *'full-length female clothes on a mannequin-light background - Stock photo ID: 688387318'*, Digital Image, <https://www.shutterstock.com/image-photo/fulllength-female- clothes-on-mannequinlight-background-688387318?src=library> accessed 28 November 2017.

Wielobob, Magdalena, *'Rose pale pink pleated two parts skirt isolated white - Stock photo ID: 672709042'*, Digital Image, <https://www.shutterstock.com/image-photo/rose-pale-pink- pleated-two-parts-672709042?src=library> accessed 28 November 2017.

studioloco, *'Beautiful young woman in colorful striped mini dress and high heels is posing with hands on hip, looking at camera and smiling. Front view. Full length studio shot isolated on white - Stock photo ID: 671345548'*, Digital Image, <https://www.shutterstock.com/image-photo/beautiful-young-woman-colorful-striped-mini-671345548?src=library> accessed 28 November 2017.

posteriori, *'womens dress on grey background - Stock photo ID: 475845745'*, Digital Image, <https://www.shutterstock.com/image-photo/womens-dress-on-grey-background-475845745?src=library> accessed 28 November 2017.

maffi, *'Gray dress isolated on white background - Stock photo ID: 543944173'*, Digital Image, <https://www.shutterstock.com/image-photo/gray-dress-isolated-on-white-background- 543944173?src=library> accessed 28 November 2017.

Karkas, *'green jacket - Stock photo ID: 56372071'*, Digital Image, <https://www.shutterstock.com/image-photo/green-jacket-56372071?src=library> accessed 28 November 2017.

Karkas, *'gray jacket - Stock photo ID: 40922188'*, Digital Image, <https://www.shutterstock.com/image-photo/gray-jacket-40922188?src=library> accessed 28 November 2017.

Karkas, *'grey woolen dress - Stock photo ID: 18450655'*, Digital Image, <https://www.shutterstock.com/image-photo/grey-woolen-dress-18450655?src=library> accessed 28 November 2017.

Ukki Studio, *'Women's jacket on a white background - Stock photo ID: 262698080'*, Digital Image, <https://www.shutterstock.com/image-photo/womens-jacket-on-white-background- 262698080?src=library> accessed 28 November 2017.

Fox, Amelia, *'Portrait of lovely woman in white shirt - Stock photo ID: 143046508'*, Digital Image, <https://www.shutterstock.com/image-photo/portrait-lovely-woman-white-shirt- 143046508?src=library> accessed 28 November 2017.

Wielobob, Magdalena, *'Flounce black skirt isolated on white - Stock photo ID: 562119286'*, Digital Image, < https://www.shutterstock.com/image-photo/flounce-black-skirt-isolated-on- white-562119286?src=library> accessed 28 November 2017.

Karkas, *'red jacket - Stock photo ID: 55538041'*, Digital Image, <https://www.shutterstock.com/image-photo/red-jacket-55538041?src=library> accessed 28 November 2017.

Maffi, *'Black skirt isolated on white background - Stock photo ID: 561852268'*, Digital Image, < https://www.shutterstock.com/image-photo/black-skirt-isolated-on-white-background- 561852268?src=library> accessed 28 November 2017.

Maffi, *'Green skirt isolated on white background - Stock photo ID: 533351494'*, Digital Image, < https://www.shutterstock.com/image-photo/green-skirt-isolated-on-white-background- 533351494?src=library> accessed 28 November 2017.

Karkas, *'gray jacket - Stock photo ID: 49412431'*, Digital Image, <https://www.shutterstock.com/image-photo/gray-jacket-49412431?src=library> accessed 28 November 2017.

Tarzhanova, 'Black female jacket with short sleeves isolated over white - Stock photo ID: 217648774', Digital Image, < https://www.shutterstock.com/image-photo/black-female-jacket-short-sleeves-isolated-217648774?src=library> accessed 28 November 2017.

Karkas, *'black coat - Stock photo ID: 61417654'*, Digital Image, <https://www.shutterstock.com/image-photo/black-coat-61417654?src=library>accessed 28 November 2017.

posteriori, *'jacket women isolated on white. with an alpha channel - Stock photo ID: 290208395'*,

Digital Image, < https://www.shutterstock.com/image-photo/jacket-women-isolated-on-white-alpha-290208395?src=library> accessed 28 November 2017.

Ksyutoken, *'Woman long jacket cloth on mannequin on white background, isolated -Stock photo ID: 526917040'*, Digital Image, < https://www.shutterstock.com/image-photo/woman-long-jacket-cloth-on-mannequin-526917040?src=library> accessed 28 November 2017.

Karkas, *'yellow coat - Stock photo ID: 151658309'*, Digital Image, < https://www.shutterstock.com/image-photo/yellow-coat-151658309?src=library> accessed 28 November 2017.

NIKS ADS, *'indian girl collage student - Stock photo ID: 729883102'*, Digital Image, < https://www.shutterstock.com/image-photo/indian-girl-collage-student-729883102?src=library> accessed 28 November 2017.

gogoiso, *'woman dress isolated - Stock photo ID: 473748049'*, Digital Image, < https://www.shutterstock.com/image-photo/woman-dress-isolated-473748049?src=library> accessed 28 November 2017.

fotosparrow, 'Female leather jacket on isolated white background - Stock photo ID: 624596366', Digital Image, < https://www.shutterstock.com/image-photo/female-leather-jacket-on-isolated-white-624596366?src=library> accessed 28 November 2017.

indira' work, *'Portrait of beautiful business woman lady style perfect body shape brunette hair wear color suit white elegance casual style secretary diplomatic protocol office uniform stewardess air hostess - Stock photo ID: 529188436'*, Digital Image, < https://www.shutterstock.com/image-photo/portrait-beautiful-business-woman-lady-style-529188436?src=library> accessed 28 November 2017.

indira's work, *'Woman model fashion style dress beautiful secretary diplomatic protocol office uniform stewardess air hostess business lady perfect body shape brunette hair wear light color suit elegance casual - Stock photo ID: 498570748'*, Digital Image, < https://www.shutterstock.com/image-photo/woman-model-fashion-style-dress-beautiful-498570748?src=library> accessed 28 November 2017.

SEMYKIN,ALEKSEI, *'Young beautiful stylish girl in white dress and black bag walking and posing outdoors - Stock photo ID: 719970826'*, Digital Image, <https://www.shutterstock.com/image-photo/young-beautiful-stylish-girl-white-dress-719970826?src=library> accessed 28 November 2017.

indira's work, *'Fashion style woman perfect body shape brunette hair wear black suit jacket pants blouse elegance casual beautiful model secretary hostess diplomatic protocol office uniform stewardess business lady - Stock photo ID: 521494879'*, Digital Image, < https://www.shutterstock.com/image-photo/fashion-style-woman-perfect-body-shape-521494879?src=library> accessed 28 November 2017.

fancy, 'Attractive young fashion model posing in the studio - Stock photo ID: 448569667', Digital Image, <https://www.shutterstock.com/image-photo/attractive-young-fashion-model-posing-studio-448569667?src=library> accessed 28 November 2017.

Karkas, 'black jacket - Stock photo ID: 93223930', Digital Image, < https://www.shutterstock.com/image-photo/black-jacket-93223930?src=library> accessed 28 November 2017.

Karkas, 'women dress - Stock photo ID: 85908295', Digital Image, <https://www.shutterstock.com/image-photo/women-dress-85908295?src=library> accessed 28 November 2017.

PhotoNAN, 'Koktel'noe dress on a model isolated on a white background - Stock photo ID: 7695052', Digital Image, < https://www.shutterstock.com/image-photo/koktelnoe-dress-on-model-isolated-white-7695052?src=library> accessed 28 November 2017.

AV_Studio, 'portrait of young woman, isolated over white background - Stock photo ID: 627315908', Digital Image, < https://www.shutterstock.com/image-photo/portrait-young-woman-isolated-over-white-627315908?src=library> accessed 28 November 2017.

hifashion, 'Evening Gown isolated with clipping path on mannequin - Stock photo ID: 117801118', Digital Image, < https://www.shutterstock.com/image-photo/evening-gown-isolated-clipping-path-on-117801118?src=library> accessed 28 November 2017.

Maffi, 'Black skirt isolated on white background - Stock photo ID: 561852151', Digital Image, < https://www.shutterstock.com/image-photo/black-skirt-isolated-on-white-background-561852151?src=library> accessed 28 November 2017.

Maffi, 'Black skirt isolated on white background - Stock photo ID: 257574199', Digital Image, < https://www.shutterstock.com/image-photo/black-skirt-isolated-on-white-background-257574199?src=library> accessed 28 November 2017.

Sermek, Gordana, 'Black elegant dress with dotted collar and sleeves, isolated over white -Stock photo ID: 580983172', Digital Image, < https://www.shutterstock.com/image-photo/black-elegant-dress-dotted-collar-sleeves-580983172?src=library> accessed 28 November 2017.

Karks, 'bkack jacket - Stock photo ID: 46843807', Digital Image, < https://www.shutterstock.com/image-photo/bkack-jacket-46843807?src=library> accessed 28 November 2017.

roberlamphoto, 'attractive female wearing beautiful jean - Stock photo ID: 39202099', Digital Image, < https://www.shutterstock.com/image-photo/attractive-female-wearing-beautiful-jean-39202099?src=library> accessed 27 October 2017.

Indiana, Diana, 'Elegant glamour woman wearing pink blouse and leggings.Urban Fashion Concept. Copy Space.Patent leather garter stockings iron leggings adult pantyhose.Sexy

Solid Black Faux Leather Leggings - Stock photo ID: 281250863', Digital Image, < https://www.shutterstock.com/image-photo/elegant-glamour-woman-wearing-pink-blouse-281250863?src=library> accessed 27 October 2017.

studioloco, *'Smiling young woman in black and white striped dress posing with hand on hip. Three quarter length studio shot isolated on white - Stock photo ID: 511921645'*, Digital Image, < https://www.shutterstock.com/image-photo/smiling-young-woman-black-white-striped-511921645?src=library> accessed 19 October 2017.

Shubinsky, Artem, *'Young businesswoman with glasses on her head - Stock photo ID: 265542326'*, Digital Image, <https://www.shutterstock.com/image-photo/young-businesswoman-glasses-on-her-head-265542326?src=library> accessed 19 October 2017.

Lexxxx, *'Beautiful young girl posing in street clothes on blue background.Isolated studio portrait - Stock photo ID: 472997485'*, Digital Image, < https://www.shutterstock.com/image-photo/beautiful-young-girl-posing-street-clothes-472997485?src=library. Accessed 19 October 2017.

PhotoMediaGroup, *'Blonde attractive woman's pink bra - Stock photo ID: 225985504'*, Digital Image, < https://www.shutterstock.com/image-photo/blonde-attractive-womans-pink-bra-225985504?src=library> accessed 3 October 2017.

Pleshakova, Katsiaryna, *'laundry icons - Stock vector ID: 173825621'*, Vector Image, < https://www.shutterstock.com/image-vector/laundry-icons-173825621?src=library> accessed 2 October 2017.

Designua, *'Structure of the Human skin. Anatomy diagram. different cell types populating the skin - Stock illustration ID: 251498023'*, Vector Image, < https://www.shutterstock.com/image-illustration/structure-human-skin-anatomy-diagram-different-251498023?src=library> accessed 29 September 2017.

Furian, Peter Hermes, *'Reflex zones of the feet - soles and side views - accurate description of the corresponding internal organs and body parts. Isolated vector illustration on white background - Stock vector ID: 318889511'*, Vector Image, <https://www.shutterstock.com/image-vector/reflex-zones-feet-soles-side-views-318889511?src=library> accessed 28 September 2017.

Majdanski, *'Smart businesswoman on the roof of the building - Stock photo ID: 184350650'*, Digital Image, <https://www.shutterstock.com/image-photo/smart-businesswoman-on-roof-building-184350650?src=library> accessed 28 September 2017.

Wittrock, Ulf, *'An image of ironing - Stock photo ID: 595621469'*, Digital Image, < https://www.shutterstock.com/image-photo/image-ironing-595621469?src=library> accessed 28 September 2017.

indira's work, 'Beautiful sexy woman wear clothes for businesswoman office style casual girl with dark hair white background fashion catalog autumn high heels lady perfect face and body makeup meeting walk - Stock photo ID: 546542413', Digital Image, <https://www.shutterstock.com/image-photo/beautiful-sexy-woman-wear-clothes-businesswoman-546542413?src=library> accessed 25 August 2017.

Coburn, Stephen, 'Pretty african american business woman at office building - Stock photo ID: 51721987', Digital Image, < https://www.shutterstock.com/image-photo/pretty-african-american-business-woman-office-51721987?src=library> accessed 14 July 2017.

Matryoha, 'female pink shoes over white - Stock photo ID: 513565996', Digital Image, <https://www.shutterstock.com/image-photo/female-pink-shoes-over-white-513565996?src=library> accessed 14 July 2017.

crystalfoto, 'Single red high heel shoe - Stock photo ID: 41388877', Digital Image, < https://www.shutterstock.com/image-photo/single-red-high-heel-shoe-41388877?src=library> accessed 14 July 2017.

Voyagerix, 'Beauty and fashion. Stylish fashionable woman wearing bright dress holding brown bag handbag, studio shot - Stock photo ID: 385215280', Digital Image, < https://www.shutterstock.com/image-photo/beauty-fashion-stylish-fashionable-woman-wearing-385215280?src=library> accessed 20 June 2017.

Undrey, 'Woman with impaired posture position defect scoliosis and ideal bearing - Stock photo ID: 265889168', Digital Image, < https://www.shutterstock.com/image-photo/woman-impaired-posture-position-defect-scoliosis-265889168?src=library> accessed 2 June 2017.

Sudowoodo, 'Female body types: skinny (underweight), fit (hourglass figure) and thick (with abdominal fat). Cute girls in underwear illustration - Stock vector ID: 417914173', Vector Image, < https://www.shutterstock.com/image-vector/female-body-types-skinny-underweight-fit-417914173?src=library> accessed 2 June 2017.

Buma, Mehmet, '3d black and white abstract spiral background with romantic heart-shaped Stock vector ID: 472362547', Vector Image, < https://www.shutterstock.com/image-vector/3d-black-white-abstract-spiral-background-472362547?src=library> accessed 2 June 2017.

opicobello, 'Color circle 12 colors - Stock vector ID: 224696710', Vector Image, <https://www.shutterstock.com/image-vector/color-circle-12-colors-224696710?src=library> accessed 2 June 2017.

Chinch, 'Woman sunglasses shapes for different women face types - square, triangle, circle, oval, diamond, long, heart, rectangle. Vector set - Stock vector ID: 490096174', Vector Image, < https://www.shutterstock.com/image-vector/

woman-sunglasses-shapes-different-women-face-490096174?src=library> accessed 23 May 2017.

Lazuin, *'Vector illustration set of various neckline types for women's' fashion. Vector in flat linear style - Stock vector ID: 641900236'*, Vector Image, < https://www.shutterstock.com/image-vector/vector-illustration-set-various-neckline-types-641900236?src=library> accessed 23 May 2017.

Phovoir, *'Portrait of a woman standing with her hands on her hips – Stock photo ID: 15972490'*, Digital Image, https://www.shutterstock.com/image-photo/portrait-woman-standing-her-hands-on-159724901> accessed 1 January 2018.

www.ingramcontent.com/pod-product-compliance
Lightning Source LLC
Chambersburg PA
CBHW061811290426
44110CB00026B/2852